THE TAI CHI SPACE

THE TAI CHI SPACE

How to Move
in Tai Chi and Qi Gong

A Pictorial Guide

Paul Cavel

The Tai Chi Space

Aeon Books

Safety note: The practice of internal energy arts such tai chi and qi gong may carry risks. The instructions and advice that follow are not in any way intended as a substitute for medical advice from an appropriately qualified physician or healthcare provider. Consult a professional before undertaking any movement, health or exercise system to reduce the chance of injury or harm. If you experience too much discomfort or pain, stop exercising immediately and consult your healthcare provider. The creators and publishers of this book disclaim any liabilities for loss in connection with following any practices, exercises or advice offered herein.

First published 2017 by
Aeon Books Ltd
118 Finchley Road
London NW3 5HT

British Library Cataloguing in Publication Data

A C.I.P. for this book is available from the British Library

ISBN: 978-1-90465-898-6

Editing and project management: Heather Cavel
Cover and interior artwork: Sophie Manham
Cover design: Sarah Lim-Murray
Edited, designed, and produced by Communication Crafts

Printed in Great Britain

www.aeonbooks.co.uk

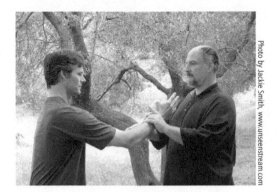

*I dedicate this book to my primary teacher, Bruce Frantzis,
without whom I could never have understood
the depths and complexity of nei gong.*

CONTENTS

ABOUT THE AUTHOR

Paul Cavel is the founder and principal of The Tai Chi Space, a London-based school established to teach Water method arts. Since 1987 Paul has studied Taoism, the *I Ching*, Five Element nei gong, medical qi gong, Yang and Wu style tai chi, Pre- and Post-birth bagua, yoga, tui na energy healing and Taoist meditation. Paul is a certified soft tissue and injury therapist (ITEC Level 4), editor of the *Inner Quest* journal and he holds a mechanical engineering certificate from London City and Guilds. He began teaching internal energy arts in 1995 with the encouragement of his primary teacher, after healing himself from a serious motorcycle accident.

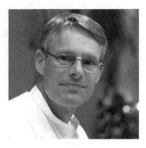

ABOUT THE ARTIST

Sophie Manham is an artist who lives and works in London.

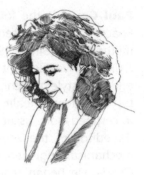

ACKNOWLEDGEMENTS

I would like to acknowledge the people who made this book possible:

My primary teacher, Bruce Frantzis, for opening my eyes to the world of nei gong, giving me the tools to initiate my personal healing journey, and for allowing me to join his bagua classes in California in the early 1990s, which changed my direction in life.

My wife, Heather Cavel, for editing, project managing and educating me in how to communicate through the written word. Without her relentless encouragement (badgering even!), this text would never have come to fruition.

Sophie Manham, the artist of the cover and interior illustrations, who put in a monumental effort to help me begin creating a visual lexicon for our internal arts peers.

Michael Mettner, who not only wrote the foreword, but whose friendship and guidance has been a continuous source of inspiration.

My good friend and fellow tai chi teacher, Jackie Smith, for his perspective and humour, and for making training a pure joy. He's taken many photos of me practising over the years, including the preceding one of my teacher Bruce and me, which I appreciate.

Oliver Rathbone for believing in me and giving me a platform to share my methodology with my internal arts peers.

Elena Moreno for inspiring the visual aspect of this pictorial lexicon, or at least the beginnings of one.

Klara and Eric King, Communication Crafts, for copyediting, interior design and production, Sarah Lim-Murray for the cover design, and the team at Aeon Books.

And to all those who have supported me and offered comments on the text, with special thanks to Jason Roberts, Sebastian Heyer, Mir Ali, Colin Hughes, Chris Binns and Nancy Maher.

FOREWORD

Michael Mettner

Our world is becoming more and more complex and is changing rapidly. Globalization and Technology are taking their toll. We are overloaded with information that we are no longer able to digest properly. Often we cannot distinguish between what is true and what is false. Our world is also becoming more and more virtual. As a result, we are losing contact with our body and with nature, nature that we are essentially a part of. All this is causing irritation, insecurity and stress.

Adding to this, many people suffer from high workloads, which today are mostly mental in nature and hence their nervous systems are burdened with stresses for which human beings are not designed. In our modern world we often experience ourselves as being helplessly exposed to circumstances we cannot change. We feel like we are losing control of our lives. All this paves the route to all kinds of stress-related disorders and illnesses, including burnout and depression.

What can we do? What would be a viable answer to these challenges?

There are many possibilities from which to choose, some more useful than others. A proven and reliable path is to learn and practise an art like tai chi. Essential aspects include relaxation, gentle movement to counter stagnation in the body, being present and becoming more and more aware of the body and its signals and needs. In this way tai chi can help practitioners heal the separation between mind and body, and reconnect to nature.

The internal arts, at least the ones solidly based on unbroken tradition, offer unique methods that can be perfectly adjusted to the needs of people. That is because Taoists, the scientists of ancient China, designed these exercise systems to enhance and coordinate the workings of mind, body and soul. Their methods of deep investigation into human existence are as of yet unparalleled by modern Western science.

Although many people practise tai chi or qi gong, it is not easy to grasp the essentials and to really reap the benefits of these internal arts. I have encountered many people who have practised tai chi for years and only regard it as some kind of "meditative" movement, without having implemented the internal principles that are essential to training.

For many years now I have worked to help executives and key players in industry leave behind burnout and stress-related illnesses, wherein the energy work of the internal arts is an important pillar. From my perspective, wasting time and effort in this way would be an inexcusable fault for my clients: when neglecting the inner principles in the internal arts, it would be better to leave them alone and just take a walk in the woods.

In this text, Paul Cavel has carved out the essential principles that make a real difference and to find appropriate ways to teach these to Westerners. He has 30 years of experience in Taoist internal arts – qi gong, martial arts and meditation. He studies with renowned teachers, the most important and inspiring being Bruce Frantzis, a Taoist Master who emphasises the Water school of the internal arts – unparalleled in the West.

For many years, Paul has been a Senior Instructor in Bruce's system without this holding him back from developing his own individual approach to training and personal development. He has taught qi gong, tai chi, bagua and meditation to thousands of students, being sensitive to the needs of individuals and always on a quest to discover the main challenges facing Westerners trying to learn Chinese internal arts, and to find even better ways to transfer his knowledge to them.

Having been Paul's student for nearly two decades, I appreciate his clear and precise style of teaching combined with a playfulness that makes learning a pleasurable experience for his students. Wherever appropriate and possible, Paul uses metaphors and pictures from everyday experiences to transmit the message.

There is a saying: "A picture tells more than a 1,000 words". That means, if chosen well, you are able to transfer an immense amount of information with a picture, unencumbered by the linear mind and providing a much clearer basis for understanding than words alone.

Metaphors, images and symbols are the language of our subconscious minds. They help to convey meaning to our consciousness and hence store in the memory quite easily and naturally. If they are chosen well, they are able to penetrate the deeper layers of our consciousness and trigger the deeply imprinted wisdom of our body. The images Paul offers can shorten the process of transmitting information, enhance our learning and awaken our bodily intelligence.

This way of teaching requires a very deep level of understanding of the material and, indeed, of human nature itself. Paul obviously has both.

The principles that follow allow the inner components of tai chi (and qi gong in general) to manifest and develop in your forms. The principles plant seeds in your mind, seeds that will be watered by practising the arts. Only then can the knowledge come alive.

This book is inspirational and a pleasure to read, and makes it easy to implement the principles, one after the other, into your internal arts practice. I recommend it to beginners as well as advanced students because, by following the instructions in this book, you will build a solid foundation for internal arts training, make your practice a lot more efficient and avoid hitting a so-called "glass ceiling" in your progress. For tai chi practitioners who want to make the best use of their valuable practice time, their lifetime and their life force, this is the book to read and to put into practice.

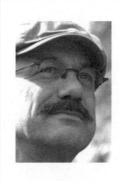 Dr Michael Mettner is an Executive Coach, Systemic Counsellor, Naturopathic Practitioner, Hypnotherapist and Internal Arts Instructor. He has more than 20 years of experience in qi gong, martial arts and various approaches to meditation. He practices near Stuttgart in Germany. www.drmettner.de

THE TAI CHI SPACE

Introduction

The allure of practising internal arts like tai chi conjures up images of a great master performing fantastic feats of speed, power and agility, one who, in all his glory and dominating force, is a virtuous sage fighting for good on his path to enlightenment, unrelenting in overcoming challenges in body, mind and spirit. Indeed, tai chi and other energy arts have been cultivated in China for millennia to produce internal power for martial arts, health, healing, and personal and spiritual development – albeit with real-life training being somewhat more pragmatic and mundane than the vision. Tai chi, an offshoot of qi gong, which fuses Taoist nei gong with Shaolin battlefield techniques and which came into being several hundred years ago, has more recently received wide acclaim in the West as an alternative approach to exercise and wellbeing.[1] When the fundamental internal content that drives and gives shape to tai chi and qi gong forms is active, both internal arts offer an effective, revitalising, slow and relaxed dichotomy to the push, force and strain mentality germane to many mainstream forms of exercise.

All Forms Are Not Created Equal

*Systems** are ideologies or schools of thought that underlie internal arts training and which make use of several to many different internal art forms.

Forms are defined by the choreography of a set of sequential movements that serve as containers for internal content to be expressed; there can be one to many different styles of any given form.

Yet anyone who considers taking up tai chi or qi gong soon finds that there are dozens upon dozens of systems, schools, forms and styles available.* The differences are not well understood in the West, where internal arts are relatively new and remain mysterious.[2] Many students train systems that have limited potential, not knowing what could be gained for the same effort and practice time simply by selecting better systems and forms to achieve their desired results. For example, most people decide to learn tai chi because of the growing body of research that supports its stress-reduction and health claims, rather than to learn how to become a skilful martial artist or to become spiritually enlightened. Martial training can indeed create a healthy body, but more as a by-product than as the prime directive of repeating fighting applications; whereas entering into the realms of meditation for spiritual development – or even just personal develop-ment – entails training that is vastly different from learning martial techniques with a relaxed or pensive state of mind, and requires a healthy body, at least to some degree,.from the outset. If you take the road to Milan with the intent of going to Madrid, the journey will be much longer than necessary, or you might not reach your destination at all; likewise, training techniques should specifically and directly develop the skills that target desired results at each stage of your development.

First and foremost, it is the internal content* that is responsible for the health, healing and power-generating benefits associated with tai chi and qi gong practice – *not forms per se.* You would not buy a car solely on the basis

> *__Internal content__ is the health and power generation techniques that energy arts, such as tai chi and qi gong, are made of.

of outward appearances without considering the mechanics under the bodywork, and forms should not be selected in this manner either. From the perspective of internal arts, like buying a car, what really counts is what happens inside the body. The ultimate aim of all energy arts training, whether you are a casual or a dedicated student, is to engage and move your insides – something that just about anyone who can stand up and walk around can develop the skill to do.*

> *And if you do want to be able to fight, you will need a healthy body as injury has taken many a seasoned professional out of the game. When their internals are active, tai chi and qi gong can keep you healthy, so you can fight another day.

Even still, in more than twenty years of teaching, I have been surprised time and again by the shocked responses I get from students when I demonstrate internal motion: that is, targeted, refined and con-trolled movement beneath the skin – whether moving fascia, ligaments, joints, bodily fluids, specific organs or the spine. The same bewildered looks emerge when I demonstrate how internal motion in one part of the body can transfer, connect to and move another part some distance away – in a student's body or in my own. Even long-term practitioners are often taken aback by the range of motion if not the depth of internal movement possible within the various forms of tai chi and qi gong.

This astonishment is the result of two self-reinforcing reasons. First, the degree to which forms are internal has been seriously downgraded in nearly all systems in the West. They essentially amount to dance choreography and yield little more than standard external exercise, which lacks the fundamental internal connections that deliver deeper health benefits. These systems are called Wushu[3] in China and are considered performance arts – not health or martial arts. Second, when learning a discipline from a foreign culture, there is a massive gap between how words translate and their actual meaning.[4] Unfortunately, many early teachers in the West have done their students a great disservice by being either unwilling or unable to teach real-deal internals, leaving lineage teachings vague and imprecise as they are passed down from one generation to the next. This is one reason why dedicated practitioners are highly concerned with lineage lines and titles: it matters who teaches you, because a person cannot share what they do not have, know or genuinely wish to transfer. As it stands, the deeper benefits associated with practice remain, by and large, elusive in the West, and the more advanced techniques that any reasonably high-level practitioner can demonstrate on demand are generally regarded as myth or fantasy.

In the early days of my training, I recall my teacher, Bruce Frantzis, demonstrating kidney breathing.[5] He allowed students to feel the movement in his lower back, as the kidneys receive a firm massage from the physical motion of the diaphragm. This basic breathing technique is fundamental to Water method arts training* since, in Chinese medicine, the kidneys are regarded as the battery pack of life, either revitalising or downgrading health and life-force energy, or what is known as qi in the East.[6] Comments from students ranged from amazement to disbelief. Those who rejected the exercise being possible, deeming the clearly visible movement as a trick or some sort of deception, created a self-fulfilling prophecy on the spot and were unlikely ever to be able to learn how to do it themselves: it is the mind, not the body, that ultimately makes anything possible. So anyone who wants to learn an art from a foreign culture – or anything new for that matter – must approach it with some degree of an open mind, albeit tempered by a healthy

*Often referred to as "Old Taoism", the **Water method** is the school of thought described by Lao Tzu in the Tao Te Ching 2,500 years ago; it is contrasted by the younger Fire method, often referred to as "Neo-Taoism", which was propagated in the Third and Fourth Centuries.

dose of scepticism, to embark on any genuine course of study and make headway along their path.

Myth Is an Image

If there is anything I have learned from my training, it is that internal arts statements are not only multi-layered, but always point to some pragmatic skill that pertains to developing the body, energy, mind or some combination of these. But how do Western students translate alien concepts into practical application? The link is metaphor.

The pages that follow are a collection of 42 principles, portrayed as illustrations and accompanied by brief explanations, aimed at conveying how the fundamental internal arts techniques function, so you can embed them and literally bring them alive in your flesh. Energy arts training does not emphasise practices for thinking about or visualising concepts. Instead, the focus is on directly experiencing what is happening inside your body – no mental projection required! But of course you must have some level of understanding of what it is you are meant to do as a starting point. Pictures can give you a means for assimilating information without simply overlaying past experiences onto concepts that are actually brand new to you.

>"Myth is an image."
>
>*Alan Watts*[7]

Images can also bypass analytical filters, allowing the mind to create new conceptual frameworks. Take cartoons as an example. Many are designed for adult entertainment and successfully continue season after season because people can take advice and even find humour in their hypocrisies from a cartoon. Most audiences would reject the same advice and narratives if offered by human beings, including by actors portraying real-life situations. Animation can function as storytelling did for the ancients, passing on cultural norms, morals and taboos from one generation to the next via the makings of myth and legend. Likewise, in order to understand the true inner workings of the internal arts, initially bypassing your mind's analytical gatekeeper allows you to discover their seemingly paradoxical logic and tap into their full potential. No equivalent applications are available in Western culture in any case, so images help to bridge the gap. One prime example is moving the body via bend-and-stretch techniques to produce circular movement rather than via reciprocal inhibition,* which, no matter how smoothly executed, can only produce linear movement.

Journey towards Unity

So why on Earth would you want to go to so much trouble to learn an ancient art from a foreign culture? First, exercise is a natural part of existence for all creatures. Watch your cat or dog the next time they wake up, and notice how they stretch and open up their body. Do you remember having to teach them how to do that? Second, there are good forms of exercise and better forms: the good forms keep you healthy and fit; the better forms heal and rejuvenate your body, energy and mind.

*Reciprocal inhibition** is the prevailing Western model for explaining how muscles control joints to move the body and states that a group of muscles on one side of a joint must contract to draw a limb towards the body while its opposing group relaxes; then the opposing group must contract while the initial group relaxes to subsequently draw the limb away from the body.

Bend-and-stretch techniques disprove this model as the only method for moving the body by activating all the body's muscles – without contraction. Just about any internal arts student who has a grounding in the basics can demonstrate this base technique on demand; truly advanced practitioners will demonstrate bend-and-stretch in every move of their flowing forms.

If you take a healthy animal, lock it in a cage and dramatically restrict its movement, in time you will notice its mood change. The animal will become depressive or aggressive and, eventually, ill – not just from a lack of exercise, but from the lack of freedom. In many ways we put ourselves in self-inflicted cages. We go from our house, to our car or public transport, to the office, to the pub or one of our favourite restaurants, and back home again. Too many people exercise very little in a day and spend a large part of it sitting and staring at screens. Bits and bytes of information transfer at lightning speed, and people cannot keep up. In comparison to our ancestors from just 100 years ago, we have become sedentary, and this lifestyle change compounds if not causes many modern illnesses.

You may not be able to slow down the pace of your life, but you can choose a form of exercise that includes targeting mental stress and tension – that which significantly impacts on how you operate your body and is ultimately responsible for your sense of wellbeing. Internal energy arts are one real answer to regaining and maintaining sanity in this rapidly advancing technological society and injecting some energy, qi, into your life.

Through the Eyes of the Ancients

The prevailing Western view is that exercise is about the muscles and the heart: that strengthening the muscles and getting the blood pumping via increased cardiovascular activity creates a healthy body. In the East, creating a healthy body starts with slow, gentle, repetitive exercise that targets and releases tension in the soft tissues and nerves, stimulates the organs, circulates blood and energy, and relaxes the body, emotions and mind. Since from an Eastern perspective organ function is associated with the emotions and governs our underlying state of health, exercise is seen as not only for the body. In fact, the concept of severance – separation of mind and body, body and emotions, energy and mind – is quite alien to Eastern thought.

You have a body and that body requires energy to live.

The more qi you have, the stronger and more vibrant you become.

Qi arts are designed to systematically and progressively release bindings that we collect throughout our lives as a result of stress, illness, injury, trauma and ageing. Tai chi and qi gong, and for that matter all internal arts, take some time and effort to learn, but the results build and exponentially multiply over time. Soft tissue techniques initially exercise the outer muscles, and they can eventually work into the deepest parts of your anatomy. As you go inside your body, layer by layer, you learn how to feel, release, open and heal all that is bound and restricted within you. In so doing, you build stamina and strengthen your body, mind and energy. Over time and with regular practice, you can manifest a body that is soft yet strong, free of restrictions and full of vitality.

A healthy body supports balanced emotions that are smooth and unsuppressed.

A calm and stable emotional state supports a mind that can be present, awake and focused.

So practice creates a positive feedback loop that reinforces balance and health on all levels of your being.

The extreme tactics of many modern exercise regimes and martial systems tend to generate a mind and emotions that are tight, hard, stress-inducing and with the mentality that something must be overcome. Internal energy arts come from the opposite approach as integrative, holistic therapies: first they seek to release, then open, balance, heal, integrate, strengthen and unify all parts into one whole.

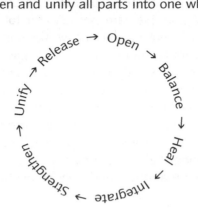

However, repeating tai chi or qi gong forms like a machine programmed with algorithms makes them lifeless and dead. Through the eyes of the ancients, energy arts were always regarded as living practices to literally wake up consciousness in the flesh and express that energy – a human being's potential – through forms that morph and develop as the individual does. Together, the 42 principles in the following pages offer a pragmatic methodology for breathing life into your forms to create lasting changes, step by step, *regardless of the specific system or external forms or styles you practise.*

How Principles Are Presented

The concepts presented here are classical principles I have learned over 30 years of dedicated internal arts training. Many are traditional, as described throughout the ages in seminal texts such as *The Tai Chi Classics,*[8] *Tao Te Ching,*[9] *I Ching,*[10] *The Book of Chuang Tzu,*[11] *The Way of Chuang Tzu*[12] and *The Inner Chapters,*[13] whereas others are my interpretations based on two decades of full-time teaching and result from my own practice and self-healing journey. All of the principles are essential components that lead a practitioner into the realm of internal exercise and bring the arts alive. Each principle has been diligently tested and yields profound and lasting results for students at all levels of experience who manage to successfully apply them in their practice.

In Parts 2 and 3 of this book, tai chi postures "contain" the internal techniques being described. Each posture serves as a good example to illustrate a specific internal principle at play, but should not be taken to mean that it is the only posture that contains the principle nor that additional principles are not relevant to any given posture. In fact, most internal principles are active throughout the entirety of tai chi and qi gong forms, and principles that have very specific applications are usually obvious and unambiguous. The purpose of showing a posture at all is to introduce relevant internal concepts in such a way that they can be brought to life in your flesh, through direct experience. This presentation is by no means an attempt to generate a dogmatic application of internal principles through a rigid system; rather, it is an attempt at offering the reader a method for gaining access to the fundamental content that drives and gives shape to internal art forms.

Three Stages for Embodying Internal Principles

Learning a tai chi or qi gong form is done piece by piece, with movements being repeated over and over again. This process allows the internals to come alive and eventually become embedded in the form, from beginning to end, without having to think about them.

The three stages of embodiment are:

First, embed the internal principle into a posture/movement that easily and naturally carries the technique due to its intrinsic design.

Second, look for the obvious places in which the internal principle can be applied elsewhere in the form.

Third, work the principle into all unobvious postures/movements of the form, until it is present and alive in your flesh throughout the entirety of the form.

Why Use Tai Chi Postures?

Although the Water method usually advocates beginning with qi gong before moving on to tai chi (a complex form of qi gong), there are several reasons why focusing on tai chi postures to learn internal content can be more useful than qi gong alone. To start with, most tai chi forms available in the West have many more postures than qi gong forms,* thereby

*This is not necessarily the case in China, where qi gong systems can include hundreds of moves, taking up to several hours to complete.

offering a wider array of possible movements to learn and train internals. Frequently repeating the same postures while layering in more internal principles can blur important distinctions essential for clarity and developing depth of skill. Second, in the West tai chi is much better known and is practised in far greater numbers than is qi gong – with the Yang style, presented here, being the most popular. That said, many forms have been downgraded from the perspective of internals or are not fully integrated, and therefore lack the content and cohesion that actually generates tai chi's deeper and more profound health and healing benefits. These principles have been practised in China for thousands of years through various internal art forms, of which tai chi is the youngest. So this is an opportunity to demonstrate what makes Chinese internal energy arts more effective forms of mind-body exercise than modern sports, forms of dance or, for that matter, external martial arts.

Visual Lexicon

This text makes use of three distinct kinds of illustration:

1. Mechanics – how forms are engineered.
2. Artistry – how forms become fluid and alive.
3. Yang style tai chi form postures – where all internal content is integrated.

Mechanics: Engineering the Form

The first stream of images deals with mechanics, offering insight into how the body physically connects up to integrate and blend within the motions of forms to create a well-oiled "machine". This is one viewpoint, like this illustration of a coin ... or is it the bottom of a bottle? It is hard to tell when viewed from a single angle only.

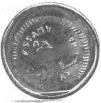

Artistry: Tapping into the Flow

The second stream of images is meant to inspire imagination and flow, to help you link with and mimic the natural world in which we live – spontaneous and always in perpetual motion. In stark contrast to mundane mechanics, it is the artistry of tai chi and qi gong that breathes life into form movements and yet relies upon them to build a solid container.

And so the object turns to the side and, with the new point of view, we see now that it is indeed a bottle. Our understanding of the bottle evolves from what was previously envisaged and hidden aspects are revealed.

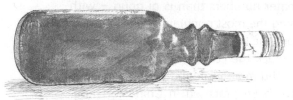

Yang Style Tai Chi Postures

The third stream of images, that of actual form postures used in tai chi and qi gong forms, introduces a movement in which the principle (from either the first or second stream) can be embedded and brought to life in your flesh.

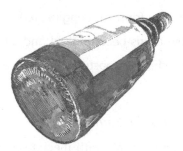

So the bottle turns to the isometric view and reveals its full depth. All three dimensions are on display, and the whole comes into focus. Only when you consider different angles can you see the complete picture, reach a deeper level of understanding and truly integrate the learning experience on more profound levels of your being.

Fusing Art and Engineering

Tai chi and qi gong fuse art and engineering, creating highly sophisticated, multi-layered, dynamic energy arts. Until practitioners grasp and balance both aspects within their forms, their practice will surely lack power and flow. People are naturally disposed to one side of the coin or the other – that is to say, more technical or artistic in their approach. In the West, we are conditioned to play to our strengths and improve individual skills. In the East, people learn to play to their weaknesses, which balances and reinforces the whole.

Only when weaknesses are strengthened can balance be achieved.

Only when balance is achieved can the realms of art and engineering be seamlessly integrated to heal, reinvigorate and maximise human potential through internal arts training.

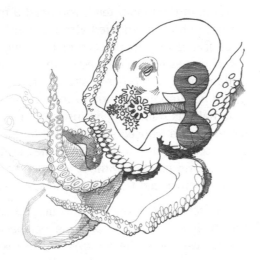

Who Can Benefit from This Book?

This book is designed to teach the fundamentals that drive and under-pin training at all levels and stages of development, not a form. There are numerous books on forms packed full of diagrams and figures that largely only serve to confuse those trying to learn tai chi and qi gong because three-dimensional motion cannot be accurately portrayed by a series of two-dimensional images; and large gaps between moves prevent students from truly following along and catching the flow. The situation is compounded by the fact that the average person's pro-prioception is distorted, leading practitioners to believe they are mimicking what they see when they might actually be doing something quite different. Anyone who has attended a tai chi class where the teacher offers corrections will have experienced this disconnect first-hand! However, for those who do not have the benefit of a teacher's live input, they can find themselves in a cul-de-sac and completely lose their way by hardwiring inaccurate movement into their bodies. These "bad habits" become hard to break later ... that is, if they manage to find a good teacher who is willing and able to offer the corrections they specifically need.

Whether you are a complete beginner, an experienced stylist or any-where in-between, learning and training an internal art always requires attuning your mind to the *modus operandi*, content and quality of the art you are practising. In the longer term, you need a method for stay-ing on track and preventing squandered effort, either by missing some of the essential principles in your practice or by trying to move on to more advanced techniques too quickly. All of the material in this book is a part of fundamental training that should never be regarded as too elementary, nor not important enough to develop and revisit time and again, as internal arts training is intrinsically circular. Through the cycling, intermediate and advanced students will find the holes in their understanding and skill set, and root out weaknesses; this guides and sets the pace for ongoing practice without a bunch of mental mumbo jumbo, allowing more advanced training to transpire organically.

Even the most advanced practitioner is encouraged to return to the basics and refine their art. In fact, from one perspective, we are all beginners. The more we know, the more we realise what we do not know. The more we accept this disposition, the more our minds can open to learning new things. As our minds open, we can see more clearly what is weak, unstable and lacks integration. I have encoun-tered too many practitioners who have put in immense effort, some over many years, in great earnest, yet their forms cannot really be considered internal. Maybe they trained a weak system, did not have a teacher who could perform or communicate internal techniques that are virtually invisible to the untrained eye, or they did not spend enough time on component practices. Whatever the case, this situa-tion is incredibly unfortunate, and, in the pages that follow, my aim is to show you how to develop quality and depth in the fundamentals, which not only unlock health and power-generating benefits but also more advanced and extraordinary levels of practice.

Creating a Practice Microcosm

Most people are only searching for a practice to maintain health and wellbeing, to prevent suffering. Even so, it takes discipline and effort to achieve, as a half-hearted attempt at practising anything once in a blue moon will yield little in return. For those who want more from their practice, it will take considerably more dedication and determination.

Whatever your level of commitment, creating your own practice microcosm is a good strategy for achieving your training goals. Take each of the principles, one thread at a time, train and develop it for several days, weeks or months, then reintegrate it back into the whole. As you cycle through and slowly upgrade each and every component, maintain a gentle intent on opening up on ever-deeper layers of your being. In time you might find you can adapt to and accommodate what might not have been conceivable before: relaxing that which is tense, strengthening that which is weak, and letting go of all that binds and restricts you from being truly free and at ease with life. There is no need to force or rush your progress in any specific way, no need for mental projections about what life will be like in the future. Instead, be content at the place where you find yourself, in the here and now, focus on creating more stability in that place and allow your next phase of development to unfurl naturally, in your own time, through accurate and sustainable practice.

PART 1

Fundamental Principles:
Nuts and Bolts

Principle 1:

Cultivate the Arts

Cultivating land is a progressive, cyclical process. The annual cycle entails ploughing, removing weeds, sowing seeds, watering, and trimming trees and carefully tending crops until the harvest, when the fruits of all that labour are enjoyed.

In the longer term, crops are rotated, compost is added to replenish lost nutrients in the soil from the proceeds of the previous year, and a careful balance between the give and take is always at play.

And the cycle repeats *ad infinitum*, always returning to the beginning and starting anew. If the land is tended with care and with the correct attitude and insight, crops can improve year after year. If the land is tended poorly, however, the quality of the harvest soon diminishes.

The internal arts are also labours of cultivation: practised to cultivate your being – that is your body, energy, mind and spirit.

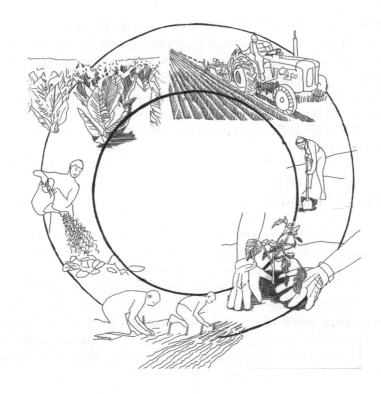

Separate and Combine

The primary tool for achieving this cultivation of art and Self is the strategy of "separate and combine", which involves separating from the whole each and every component of the arts, practising and singularly embedding them in your being, then reintegrating them into the whole again. This process allows you to see each thread clearly and in its own light.

Without this directive, the various threads of the internal arts cannot become fully activated, which diminishes overall results. If each thread is weakened by not being properly developed, the synergy that occurs from ongoing training cannot possibly yield the health and longevity that is promised. So the wise student separates and combines all the individual components of internal exercises in a never-ending cycle – continuously and meticulously deconstructing and rebuilding forms anew.

Cyclic Training

The internal energy arts are famous for their application of circles, and they show up in the very spirit of training. Why? Because human beings operate in cycles, one of the most fundamental and influential of which is the four seasons. We have an intrinsic need for repetition and reinforcement; the willingness to return to the beginning again is perhaps equal to if not more important than advancing learning and self-development. So training yields the best results when attuned to our individual and natural cycles, allowing practice to evolve and adjust to both internal and external changes.

However, a circle has no beginning and no end. So, from the perspective of the Water method, you can never really return to exactly from where you came, because you, as a human being, fundamentally change as the result of your life experience – of which practice can be an integral part. But the emphasis is on the return, the deliberate act of revisiting everything that you trained before, from the most basic techniques to the most profound, over and over again in shorter and longer training cycles. By revisiting fundamental components, practice is kept fresh and alive, enabling ever deeper insights as you delve through the layers of your body, mind and qi.

Moving only forwards is a linear progression. By contrast, cyclic training transforms into a spiral, with each rotation taking you deeper into yourself and closer to your core, allowing you to uncover new meanings and gain greater clarity. And so one of the functions of the spiral reveals itself: slowly, over time, through repetition of the same techniques and principles being applied again and again, you

refine your art,

sink deeper into yourself,

assimilate the various and seemingly paradoxical aspects of both your training and yourself, and

realise more of your true nature.

Principle 2:

The Rule of Thirds

The Rule of Thirds states that if you are healthy and not compromised in some way, use two-thirds of your energy and effort while always leaving one-third in reserve.

If you are compromised in some way, especially if ill or injured, practise the opposite: never use more than one-third of your energy or effort, and always keep two-thirds in reserve.

When pushed beyond their comfortable limits, the body, mind and qi become strained and trigger the body's instinctual self-defence mechanisms. When activated, the nervous system pulls all parts of the body towards its centre to prevent damage.

When the nerves tighten,
the muscles harden,
blood and qi circulation constricts,
and the body learns to distrust the mind, keeping your system on "red alert".

Whereas maintaining one-third in reserve and not overloading your system is precisely what allows:

The nerves to relax.
The muscles to let go.
Stretches to sink deeper into your body.
The space in your body to open up.
Blood and qi to flood the body.
Total mind-body-qi nourishment.

This principle is the guiding rule for all training, in terms of which practices you train, when and for how long to ensure positive results in all aspects of your development.

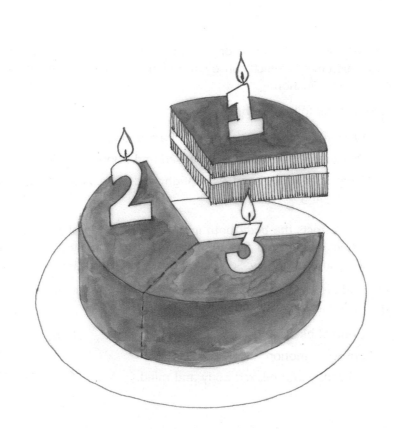

Principle 3:

Become Sung

Finding the middle way is one of the goals of internal arts training, to avoid extremes – which cause stress and tension, or slow and sluggish body-mind function.

Contrast the following three postures:

Western military posture: tense, hard and stiff. Too yang.

Western relaxed posture: collapsed and floppy. Too yin.

Sung: soft and relaxed, yet upright and open. A good balance of yang and yin.

Tension restricts the body, both internally and externally. But when the body goes floppy and flimsy, this too restricts bodily functions, especially blood and qi flow. So relaxed doesn't mean collapsed!

The middle way – *sung* – is open, relaxed and unbound, encouraging the body into an easy, upright posture for:

Optimal blood and qi flow.

Effortless motion.

A healthy and relaxed body and mind.

Too yang   Too yin   Balanced
                                   yin and yang

Principle 4:

Build the Pyramid of Giza

... Not the Leaning Tower of Pisa!

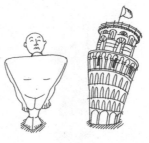

Western military posture: feet together, knees locked, chest forward and raised, shoulders back, chin up and arm muscles engaged. This stance produces a top-heavy, narrow foundation, which is rigid and unstable.

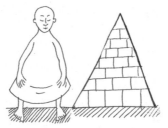

Eastern internal arts posture: feet shoulders' width apart, knees bent, pelvis dropped, chest, shoulders and face sink downwards, spine raised and arms relaxed. This stance produces a light top (from roughly above the waistline to the crown of the head) and a heavy bottom (from below the waistline to the feet), and thereby a relaxed and stable foundation.

11 Steps to Good Posture

Proper postural alignments can be achieved in an 11-part, sequential process, working from the bottom up, then from the top down.

1. The feet are about shoulders' width apart – not less, but a little more is okay – and the toes point forward. The knees are roughly the same width apart as the feet.

2. The knees are bent but do not protrude forward of the toes. Begin with locked knees, then unlock and bend them just enough for the thighs to engage. When done correctly, the centre of the knee is over the centre of the arch of the foot. This is the correct postural alignment each and every time the knees bear weight.

3. The pelvis is relaxed and hangs off the spine. The back of the pelvis descends, which must be done without pushing the knees further forward or allowing any pressure to build up in the knees. The descent is generated by letting go of the lower back muscles, which releases the back of the pelvis to gravity. The pressure from this gentle releasing action transfers to the feet.

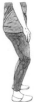

4. The spine rises in two distinct stages:

    » First, pluck up your back, so the rising spine gently yet firmly lifts and extends all the way from the lumbar spine up to the top of the back/base of the neck (T1–C7).[14] *There is no hardening or tensing whatsoever.*

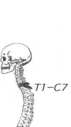

T1–C7

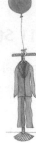

» Second, the neck is empty – although not weak or floppy – with a soft, gentle rising in the spine through the neck all the way up to the skull. It is the rising in the neck that takes out any slack, like a helium balloon takes out the slack of a string when attached from below.

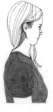

5. To align the lumbar and thoracic spine correctly:

    » Stand with your spine touching the edge of something, such as a door, so that the prop is not in contact with your gluteal muscles (bottom) or shoulder blades.

    » Make sure your legs are aligned correctly and you do not lean or rest your weight against the prop.

    » Smoothly drop the back of the pelvis.

    » Then, if need be, gently draw the lumbar spine backwards.

    » Raise T1–C7 up and back, so that the bulk of your lumbar-thoracic spine is simultaneously touching the prop without pressure, either internally or externally. There is no expectation for your cervical vertebrae and skull to touch the prop, so don't force the head and neck in any way. The main goal is to align the spine plumb vertical and obtain the straightest possible lumbar-thoracic spine – without igniting any sense of strain.

    Practising this sequence from time to time will allow you to check your spine alignment as well as your progress.

6. The head draws slightly up and backwards, so that the centre of the head moves towards the centre of the torso and pelvis – again without igniting any sense of strain. The face drops, so that the centre of the eye and ear are level on the horizontal plane.

7. The tip of the tongue makes light contact with the hard palate just behind the top row of teeth and remains in this position throughout the entirety of your practice, to link an important qi flow in the human body – the microcosmic orbit. The rest of the tongue stays completely relaxed.

8. The chest and shoulders are relaxed and drop down without collapsing or bending the spine. As they sink, they draw down energy into the belly and hips, thereby beginning the emptying of the upper body.

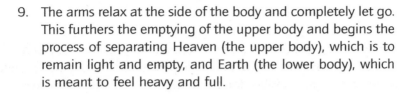

9. The arms relax at the side of the body and completely let go. This furthers the emptying of the upper body and begins the process of separating Heaven (the upper body), which is to remain light and empty, and Earth (the lower body), which is meant to feel heavy and full.

10. As you stand, continuously raise the spine from *ming men*,* while continuously dropping the back of the pelvis. Whenever you adjust your spine, follow by releasing and relaxing your face, shoulders, arms, chest, belly, back muscles and tailbone. The more you develop skill with this slow, incremental release, the deeper you can plunge your root into the earth, and the more blood and qi you will circulate.

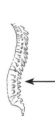

***Ming men** is an energetic point in the lumbar spine directly opposite to the lower tantien.
The **lower tantien**, a nonphysical space centrally located below the navel, is where the upper body and lower body separate and meet; it is the junction for all the energy channels that affect physical health and vitality.

11. **Safety note:** don't strain the occipital area (where the skull meets the top of the neck) by applying too much strength to the rising of the neck. Relax the neck and hold up the body from T1–C7. Don't let pressure build in the lower spine or knees by sinking down too strongly. You can gently raise the spine to release the pressure. Always adhere to the Principle of Thirds when making postural adjustments to avoid injury and encourage maximum blood and qi flow.

Principle 5:

Breathe with the Diaphragm

Breathing in tai chi and qi gong is centred deep in the belly and fully activates the diaphragm, a dome-shaped sheet of internal skeletal muscle that is responsible for breathing.[15] There are many levels to breathing practice, with each layer relying on the previous one to take root and yield results.

However, what is important in the beginning is to spend a considerable amount of time cultivating a smooth, regular, deep and balanced breath — without sudden gasps or holding the breath between inhaling–exhaling or exhaling–inhaling.

Many practitioners make the mistake of forcing their breath to coordinate with form movements, which ultimately leads to closing down the breath and generating more tension. You don't want to fix your breath to the rhythm of your form in any way.

> Let the breath be natural and easy without igniting any sense of force or strain in body or mind.

When you breathe poorly or into the upper chest, the lower organs stagnate, the mind drifts and bodily functions, such as blood circulation and digestion, are weakened. Autonomic nerve signals are responsible for these changes and respond to sensory information about whether the body is under stress, or more or less in a relaxed state.

> When you breathe well and into the belly:
> the nerves discharge and enhance bodily functions;
> the body lets go and opens up;
> sung is amplified; and
> circulation and presence improve.

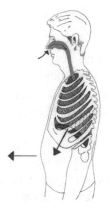
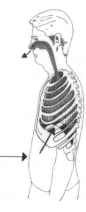

In-breath −
diaphragm descends, belly swells

Out-breath −
diaphragm rises, belly releases

When practised correctly, there is very little or no rising and falling
of the rib cage (chest)

Principle 6:

The Mind's Focus

The mind leads the body in practice. If the mind is not focused, practice is poor, and potential results are greatly diminished.

> When you dream, visualise or space out, you do not have any awareness of what you are doing in the here and now.

> Whereas, if you are present and in the moment, your mind can focus on the matter at hand, and even a short practice can be incredibly productive.

Stop and take a break if your focus becomes forced, tense or tight in any noticeable way, or the body will soon follow, and your energy will wane. Some days you might have to accept that you must do less.

Your focus wants to remain soft, relaxed and continuous throughout the entirety of your practice to cultivate the energy, vitality and health for which the internal arts are famous.

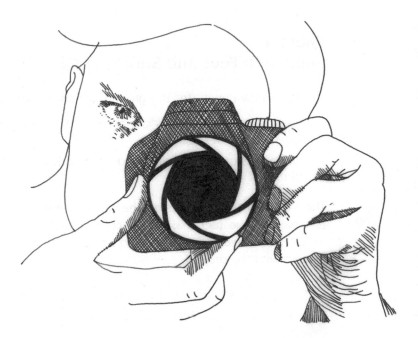

Principle 7:

Grow Your Root

Phase 1:
Plant Your Feet and Sink Your Qi

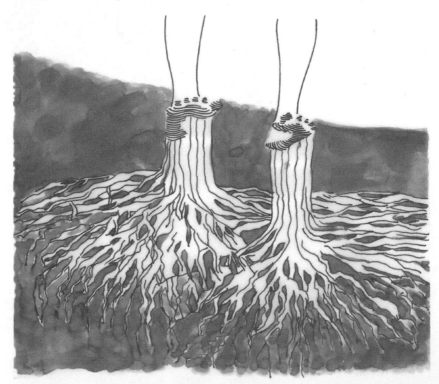

Sinking energy penetrates the ground and establishes your root.

> Poor postural alignments create excess tension in the muscles and prevent qi from sinking.

> Proper postural alignments allow the body and mind to relax and qi to sink.

The weight of the body sits on the feet, while the heels, outside edges and balls of the feet make solid contact with the ground. Keep the arches of the feet from collapsing as they remain free from making contact with the ground.

To plant a tree, you dig a hole and bury the roots. In tai chi and qi gong, your energetic roots grow out of the soles of your feet as your qi sinks down – no digging required!

Align your body,
　　　　relax your muscles,
　　　　　　　sink your qi, and
　　　　　　　　　　grow your root.

Phase 2:
Release Tension to Develop Your Root

Sinking is an act of letting go. (Let that sink in!)

Gravity pulls objects down, so when you place a stone just below the surface of the water, you can watch it sink down to the bottom as you let go.

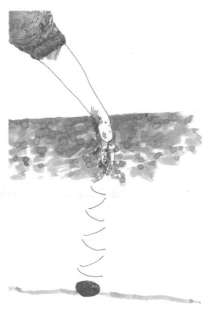

First sink your qi to establish your root, then let your practice become deeper.

In tai chi and qi gong, relaxation is cultivated by systematically letting go of tension and slowly working deeper towards your core. Start at the top of your head and sink any tension you feel down your body, out of your feet and into the earth, like a bath emptying of water. Slowly work downwards (never go up!), releasing any tension you find en route.

As you are able to let go into the earth more and more, you will become freer, more open and alive. This process not only releases your body and circulates your qi, but also develops your root.

Principle 8:

Moving in Three-Dimensional Space

The three planes of all internal arts motion are:[16]

Transverse – horizontal plane

Sagittal – front–back–vertical plane

Coronal – left–right–vertical plane

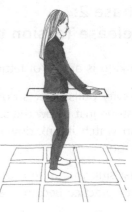

Transverse plane

The three axes of motion in engineering are:

X axis

Y axis

Z axis

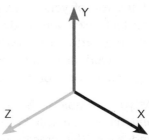

Both describe motion in three dimensions and provide a framework for how to move in the space around you.

Internal arts forms are always practised in all three dimensions, otherwise connectivity throughout the body and depth of motion will be limited or lost. When lost, internal content cannot manifest in your form, and practice is dramatically downgraded.

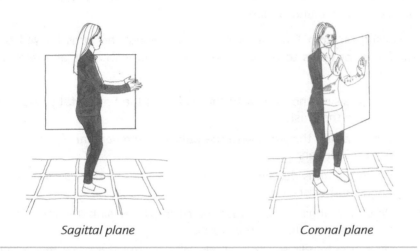

| Sagittal plane | Coronal plane |

Some practitioners believe that if they only practise their form accurately, internal content will naturally come alive. To some degree, this is true. So pay attention to detail, specifically with respect to how movements use three-dimensional space.

Tai chi and qi gong forms serve as containers for internal content:

> If a container is weak, it does not contain.
>
> The contents that the container contains are the internal techniques that generate the deeper health and healing benefits associated with tai chi and qi gong practice.

Principle 9:

Arms Are Led by Hands and Wrists

Sung, an open and unbound state, is the underlying quality of all motion in tai chi and qi gong.

Following on from Principle 3 to generate sung, the arms are led by the hands or wrists to allow the rest of the arms to relax and release to gravity.

> When raising the arms with the palms on the horizontal plane, lift from the wrists.
>
> When raising the arms with the palms on the vertical plane, lift from the fingers.
>
> When the arms descend with the palms up, sink the backs of the hands and wrists.
>
> When the arms descend with the palms down, sink the heels of the palms and front of the wrists.
>
> When the hands rise and fall, the elbows and shoulders sink at all times – even if the elbows physically rise in space. *The shoulders never rise.*
>
> The spine rises and the chest sinks at all times. It is the spine that holds up the body.

These points of reference will allow you to use minimal effort while moving without collapsing and, in so doing, deepen sung.

When raising the arms:

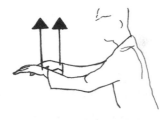

*Wrists rise with palms on
the horizontal plane*

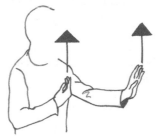

*Fingers rise with palms on
the vertical plane*

When sinking the arms:

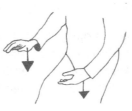

*When the palm is up, sink the
back of the hand; when the palm
is down, sink the heel of the palm*

When raising and sinking the arms:

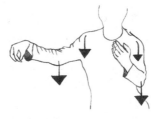

*Elbows and shoulders sink
at all times*

Principle 10:

Create Circular Motion

Circularity is systematically cultivated through internal arts training.

Central to the Principle of Circularity, from the perspective of the body, is not locking the limbs, which can only generate superficial stretching. Maintaining a bend in the limbs allows continuity of motion and deeper stretching to take place that, together, enable access to your insides.

So the first rule of circularity is to avoid locking the limbs, which creates:

Straight lines.

Disconnection from your insides.

Tension and rigidity.

Reduced blood and qi flow.

A locked limb also breaks the flow of your form and causes inertia.

The subject of circularity is pervasive and deep in internal arts training, with many layers of refinement. In the beginning, the key is to always keep your arms and legs bent – yet never to their maximum bend either. Too much bend generates the same negatives as a locked limb.

A straight limb generates a linear force.

A bent limb generates a circular force.

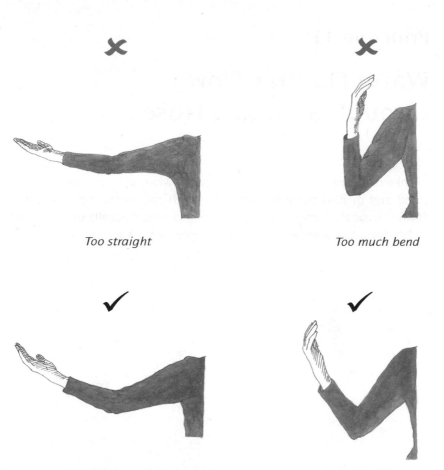

Too straight

Too much bend

Two-thirds straight

Two-thirds bent

When the limbs are kept within the range of the Rule of Thirds, which is two-thirds bent or two-thirds straight:

The muscles release.

Fascia, the body's connective tissue, is engaged.

Bend-and-stretch, a relaxation-based motion, is activated.

Reciprocal inhibition, a tension-based motion, is diminished and eventually eliminated.

Circularity, and therefore continuum, are engaged.

Blood and qi circulate more powerfully, and you cultivate your life-force energy.

Principle 11:

Water Doesn't Flow through a Kinked Hose

A kinked hose reduces water flow. Likewise, when the muscles contract, blood and qi flow become restricted, which causes the body to close down. The goal of internal arts practice is to systematically open up the body's pathways and get the fluids and energy flowing optimally again.

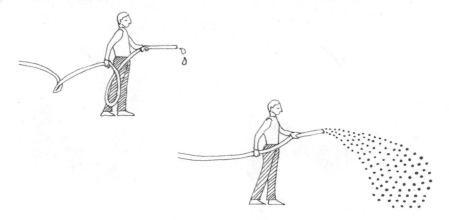

Sung, an unbound state, is the underlying quality of all tai chi and qi gong training, that which enables an open system free from residual and daily tensions. So whatever level of practice you engage in, whether component practices in this section or a fluid tai chi or qi gong form:

> Look for habitual contractions and set a relaxed intent on letting go and releasing them in each posture, in every transition and in all body parts – external and internal.
>
> Eradicate bindings,
>> release tension,
>>> prevent contractions, and
>>>> open up and let go
> ... to enable blood and qi to flood and nourish your body.

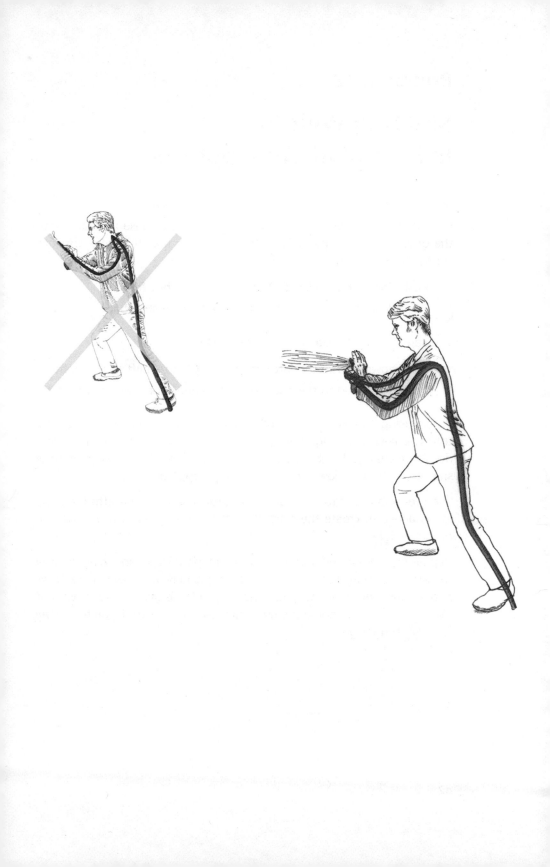

Principle 12:

Shifting Weight Is Like Walking Upstairs

In order to walk upstairs, you push off one leg to raise and step with the other. Weight shifts in tai chi and qi gong use this same effort to shift forward and back.

Push down and back with the back leg to shift forward.

Push down and forward with the front leg to shift back.

The same is true for side-to-side weight shifts.

Push down and to the left with the left leg to shift to the right.

Push down and to the right with the right leg to shift to the left.

When using this method to shift weight in any direction, make sure that you keep your alignments, and that your pelvis remains level and does not change height. There is no up and no down; the motion is smooth, even and slow – never sudden, choppy or fast.

Set a relaxed intent to maintain an unbroken, continuous effort. As one leg is active to create the shift, the other leg is passive to receive the body's weight.

Repeating weight shifts as a component practice is an excellent way to target tension in the lower body, especially the lower back, hips and thighs. You can slowly unwind and release stuck tissues without more complicated choreography, which can reduce your ability to stay focused and let go.

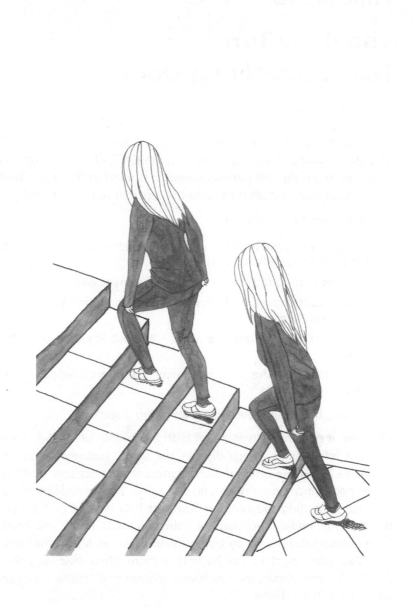

Principle 13:

The Body Turns Like a Revolving Door

The body turns from the centreline of your body, with the motion initiated by the waist. If turning to the left, the left half of your body moves back, and the right half moves forward; if turning to the right, the right half of your body moves back, and the left half moves forward.

While the waist turns the body:

> The knees remain stable – without any sideways motion (slightly forwards or back is natural).
>
> The feet remain rooted – without rolling in or out.
>
> Your qi continuously sinks – without disconnecting from the legs or excessively rising.
>
> The upper body follows the waist – without any twisting in the spine.
>
> The arms follow the torso – reducing the effort needed to practise your forms.

In this way, the torso moves like a revolving door.

However, if movement is initiated with a shoulder or by the chest, the pelvis is left behind, which distorts the spine. Likewise, if movement is initiated with the arms or hands, strength and tension build in the upper body, once again distorting the spine. Both scenarios make you top-heavy, creating the Leaning Tower of Pisa instead of the Pyramid of Giza! Remaining conscious of your two-thirds effort will keep you from creating distortions by trying to turn too far. Many students find that their turns must reduce by half or more when reviewing the simple checkpoints above, as they reveal tension and "sticky" or restricted soft tissues in the body.

Turning back and forth as a component practice is a great way to target tension in both the upper and the lower body, allowing you to unwind and release it from your body without more complicated choreography reducing your ability to stay focused and let go.

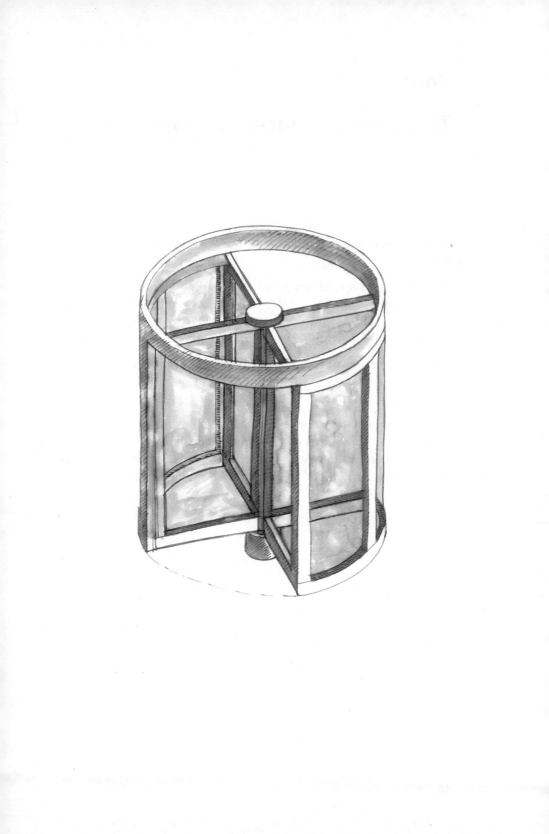

Principle 14:

The Down Creates the Up

In a pulley system, a rope is looped over a wheel, so when you pull down on one side, the other side rises, with gravity assisting the lift instead of diminishing it.

In many tai chi and qi gong movements, one arm descends while the other arm rises. To activate the pulley system in your practice, always initiate with the downwards force. By doing so, the downwards force in one arm can activate the rising of the other – with very little effort.

Generating an upwards motion with the downwards force, traditionally referred to as "the down creates the up", is key to both connected body motion and energy conservation.

This foundational principle is the basis of more subtle and refined techniques to come, so focus on the descending half of the cycle early on in your training to develop connectivity and sensitivity. Later, you will apply your skill to unlock more advanced internal techniques.

Visualise a Puppet on a String

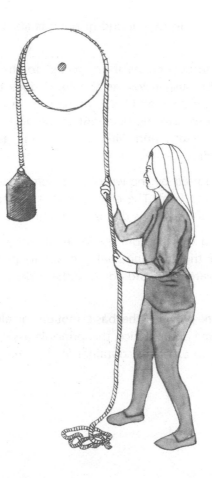

Principle 15:

Move Like a Puppet on a String

The basic motion in tai chi and qi gong is like that of a puppet on a string.

The head is suspended as if connected to the sky, but there is no strength in the suspension as the head does not lift up the body: rather, the spine does at T1−C7, as covered in Principle 4. The lifting is just enough to take the slack out of the neck, like a helium balloon rising, ever so gently and without employing any upwards muscular force of its own.

The arms are raised by the wrists or fingers, allowing the hands to be empty, open and light. The elbows and shoulders release downwards with the flow of gravity, as discussed in Principle 9.

When raising a leg, lift from the knee, allowing the foot to hang and relax. Fold in the hip (inguinal groove) to prevent the pelvis from tipping backwards, forwards or to either side, as well as to maintain balance.

This framework provides the basic motion for all tai chi and qi gong forms. With time and practice, this principle assists in manifesting sung and serves as an excellent container for all other internal content.

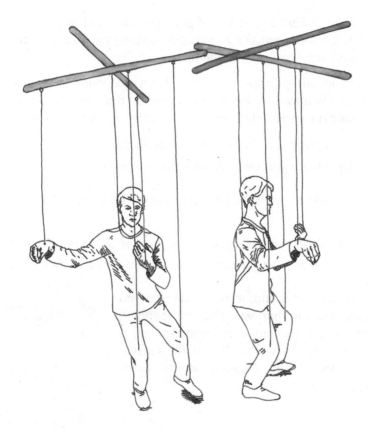

Principle 16:

Don't Play the Juggler

If you jump from one aspect of practice to another or try to cram in too much too soon, practice becomes a juggling act, and you are likely to drop all, not just some, of the balls.

Focus on one principle at a time for a minimum of several practice sessions in a row. In this way, you deepen the experience and benefits by building a solid platform, while rooting out weaknesses.

Each piece you skip over weakens all others.

Each piece you embody improves the whole.

Work slowly through the principles, and don't be in a rush to reach the end.

To have an end in sight, the mind must act with a linear force.

The internal arts are circular in nature, and a circle has no end.

Go round and round, revisiting all that you enjoy and all that you do not, spending time with each component and working it deeper into the whole. This is the circular methodology of learning, which yields lifelong, positive results.

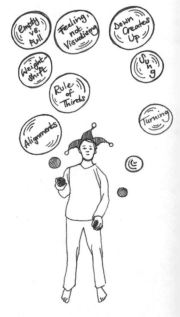

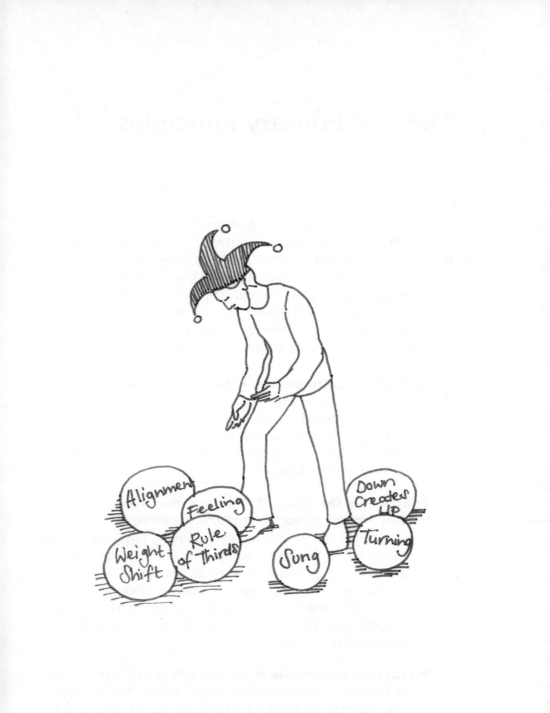

The Five Primary Principles

Of all the internal principles – both those presented in and those beyond the scope of this text – five threads are essential for developing and weaving together before all others. They are so fundamental that most practitioners skip over them with very little thought. However, they not only serve as the building blocks for your foundation, but also become the very vehicle through which your practice can reach new heights. So without these five principles, tai chi and qi gong forms cannot really be considered internal.

Principle 1: Cultivate the Arts in circular fashion, otherwise progress is always linear and never returns to the beginning to refine individual threads in relation to all others, which builds in a glass ceiling. In tandem with "separate and combine", circular learning is the prime directive of internal energy arts and yields genuine advancement.

Principle 2: The Rule of Thirds is the single most important principle in the Water method, enabling practitioners to advance at the fastest rate by preventing injury and arousal of the body's protective, safety mechanisms. When the body is pushed beyond its natural limits, the nerves counter: both internal and external range of motion is blocked, mind-body trust is severed and either progress is stunted or the practitioner can too easily be completely taken out of the game by injury or internal resistance.

Principle 3: Become Sung. The first goal of tai chi and qi gong is to relax as tension inhibits blood and qi flow, but relaxed doesn't mean collapsed. Maintaining a relaxed upright posture encourages the nervous system, the whole body, its qi and the mind into a state of deep letting go.

Principle 4: Postural Alignments build the container of your form. Lao Tzu discusses the importance of the hole in the middle of the wheel, without which the wheel cannot turn, and the usefulness of the empty cup, which can receive content.[17] So, in a real and direct sense, it is the internal space generated by postural alignments that provides the framework to embody all other internal principles.

Principle 10: Create Circular Motion rather than using conditioned reciprocal inhibition to move. The alternating bend-and-stretch rhythm in the soft tissues creates circular motion and is the doorway to internal exercise, the bedrock of all other motion in the internal arts. This is the first principle that directly speaks to integrated, whole-body movement, which is why it does not follow the sequence.

Always keep these five principles in mind and allow them to guide your training no matter how advanced or deep your practice becomes.

PART 2

Internal Principles for Connectivity and Flow

Principle 17:

Warm Up Body and Mind

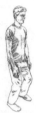

When beginning any form of exercise, the initial objective is to warm up the body and focus the mind on the task at hand. When done sufficiently and accurately, the body and mind are prepared for a greater range of motion and more vigorous activity, thereby preventing strain and injury, and maximising potential results. This is especially true when compromised and for the elderly.

Beginning Form

Beginning Form is exactly what it says: beginning the form, the first movement of tai chi.

Repeating this exercise between five and 20 times before flowing through the whole form:

> Releases physical and mental tension.
> Stretches the soft tissues (fascia, muscles, tendons and ligaments).
> Lubricates the joints.
> Initiates more powerful circulation of blood and qi.
> Draws the mind into the body.
> Engages whole-body motion.

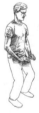

Now you can maximise potential results and benefits from your practice.

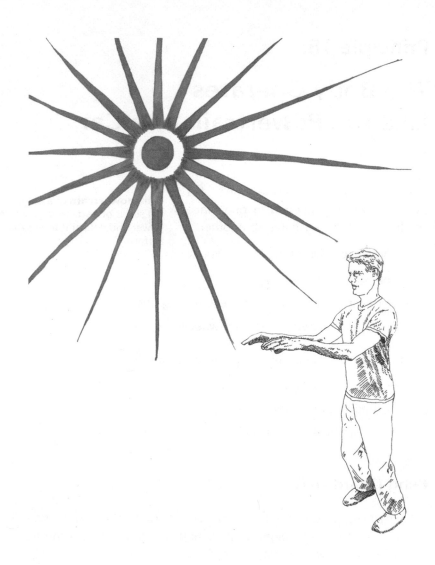

Beginning Form is a high-yield movement. I often use it in qi gong courses to teach motion on the vertical plane while building in specific fundamental principles like sung and the Rule of Thirds.

Repeating Beginning Form in a continuous loop gives tai chi practice a touch of qi gong flavour, which is repetitive in nature, allowing the practitioner to embody various layers of internal content by bringing them alive in the flesh and then carrying them forward throughout the form.

Principle 18:

The Body Operates Like the Powertrain of a Car

The body acts like the powertrain* of a car as power is generated in one place yet directed and transferred to another.

*The **powertrain** of a car is the series of parts that generate power and deliver it to the road surface.

From the perspective of the car, power is:

>generated in the engine,

>>directed by the steering mechanisms, and

>>>transferred to the road wheels.

From the perspective of the human body, power is:

>generated in the legs,

>>guided by the waist, and

>>>applied through the arms and hands.

Peng (Ward Off)

The First Peng posture begins the process of linking three fundamental components (shifting weight, turning and the down creates the up – Principles 12, 13 and 14, respectively), so that:

>the legs become the primary driver of the movement,

>>the waist becomes secondary by receiving, guiding and amplifying power from the legs,

>>>which is applied through the arms and hands.

Now whether that power is for health, healing, longevity or martial arts, it's all one power – qi! It is the practitioner who decides on which application(s) to focus and develop.

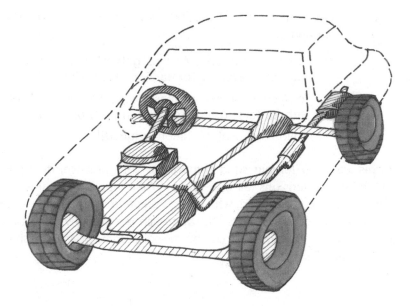

Principle 19:

Soften to Close, Release to Open

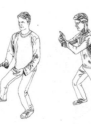

The basic rhythm of the form is to follow the natural flow of yin and yang.

> To close – the body softens, gathers and absorbs without tension or contraction of any kind.

> To open – the body releases, stretches and expands without force or excess effort in body or mind.

> ... No reciprocal inhibition required!

In this way, you remain sung throughout your practice, dredging up and releasing tensions as you train. When applied accurately, the vascular system is engaged, which takes pressure off the heart, yielding low-impact vascular exercise. This approach is especially important for anyone who is ill, injured or compromised in some way, or wishing to heal old injuries.

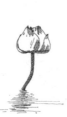

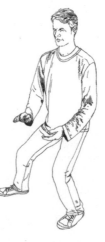

Lu (Roll Back) and Ji (Press)

Lu and Ji are pure yin and yang, respectively, and therefore are an excellent pair for working with the concept of soften to close and release to open.

> To close, first you must be open, which is the case in the previous posture of Peng.

> Next comes the smooth transition into Lu as you soften, gather and absorb.

> In Ji, smoothly and continuously release, stretch and expand to open.

Soften to close and release to open is how to harmonise with the natural flow of yin and yang like a flower that closes at dusk and opens at dawn.

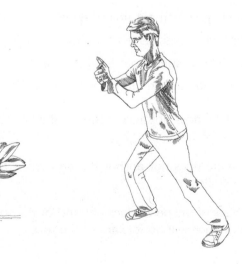

Principle 20:

The Body Makes Use of Anchors

The body uses a series of anchors to prevent distortions in postures caused by overextensions. These stable points keep in place specific parts of the body while allowing the next part in the chain to stretch out free of distortion.

In this way, the stretching of the soft tissues goes deeper into the body, where the insides can be accessed with less effort and greater relaxation:

The feet anchor the legs.

The back of the pelvis anchors the spine.

The spine anchors the arms.

The elbows anchor the hands.

In tandem with the Rule of Thirds and the Principle of Circularity, anchors guide all tai chi and qi gong movements, so that:

The legs stretch out from the feet.

The spine stretches out from the legs.

The elbows stretch out from the spine.

The hands stretch out from the elbows.

If the elbow does not anchor the hand when the hand is extended, the elbow will lock.

If the spine does not anchor the arm when the arm is extended, the spine will distort.

If the back of the pelvis does not anchor the spine as you shift forward, the front knee will go forward of the toes.

If the feet do not anchor the legs, the feet will roll, and you lose your alignments, root and balance.

An (Push)

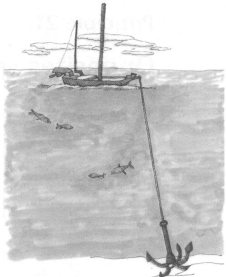

The posture of An presents a balanced dichotomy with one simple weight shift and push

without turning,

without stepping, and

without added, unnecessary complexity.

Practice An with smoothness, continuum and grace.

Start by anchoring your feet and, in one wave, from bottom to top, sequentially and fluidly anchor the pelvis, then spine, and finally the elbows.

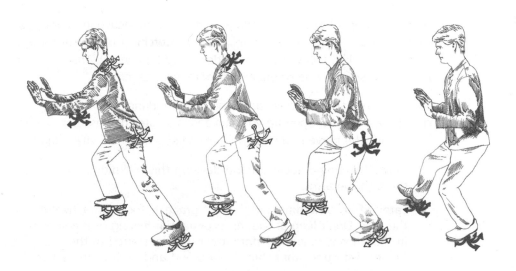

Principle 21:

Opposites Spread Open the Body

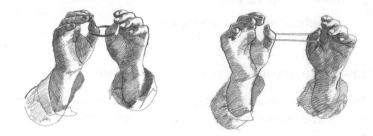

When an arm extends in one direction and the other arm extends in the near-opposite, while adhering to the Principle of Circularity, the body stretches out on a profound level like an elastic band drawn out from both ends.

Single Whip

In the final opening of Single Whip, both arms are active in near opposition to each other to generate a deep stretching of all the body's soft tissues (skin, facia, muscles, tendons and ligaments). This action is known as "split" – one of the eight energies of tai chi.

Through this action, while adhering to the Principle of Thirds, you gain access to and open up your insides, activate the vascular system, stretch out the nerve pathways and create space for the vital organs.

> In the beginning, focus on and develop this technique only through the arms.

> Later, after some time and diligent practice, focus on activating the legs. Don't leap ahead: an experiential feeling of the stretch in the arms is required before it can be transferred to the legs free of distortions that shut down blood and qi flow and sever your root!

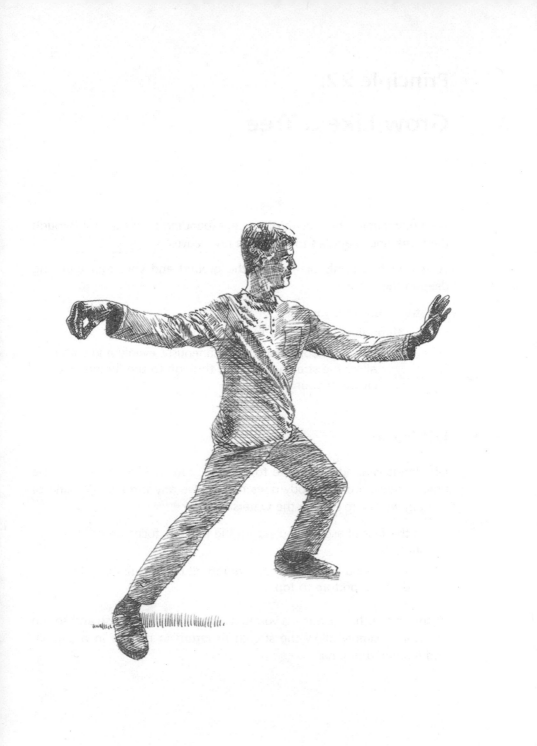

Principle 22:

Grow Like a Tree

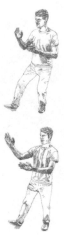

The body mimics the growth of a tree, expanding from the root through the trunk and branches to the twigs and leaves.

With your feet firmly planted on the ground and your root plunging deep in the earth:

> stretch up from your feet;
>
>> through your legs and torso; and,
>>
>>> in one smooth wave, simultaneously, evenly and softly allow the stretch to extend through to the fingertips and crown of your head.

Lift Hands

Lift Hands is an ideal posture to practise growing like a tree since the final expansion of the body does not involve any turning, stepping or shifting weight to muddy the waters.

> In the first phase, as you set up the posture, focus on generating sung.
>
> In the second phase, stretch through all the soft tissues of the body, from bottom to top.

At the end of the posture, as you move into the next release and soften everything, simply allow the stretch to return to neutral in a smooth and regulated manner.

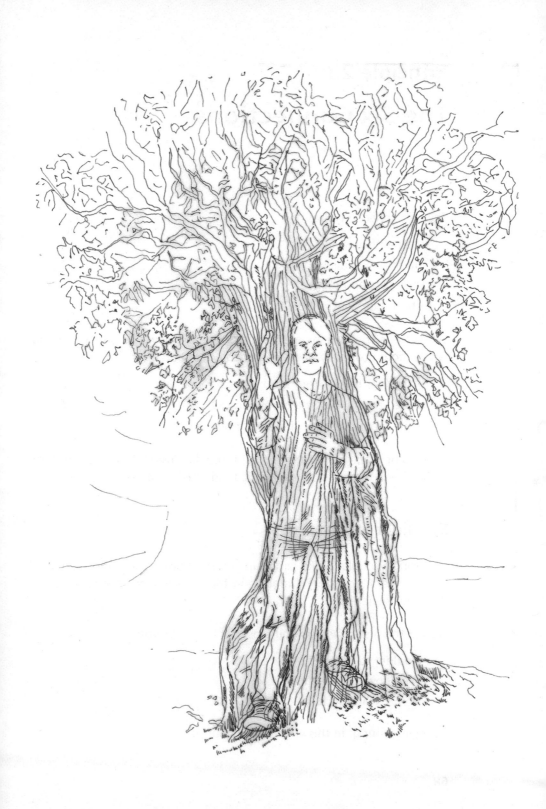

Principle 23:

The Six Connections

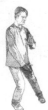

The six connections are:

> the hands and feet,
> elbows and knees,
> shoulders and hips

... on both sides of the body.

When these connections are forged, the body moves as one integrated whole, both physically and energetically, so that:

> If the foot moves, the hand moves.
> If the knee moves, the elbow moves.
> If the hip moves, the shoulder moves.

Movement can be external, in three-dimensional space, and/or internal – in the soft tissues, joints, fluids and qi of the body.

Shoulder Strike

Practising Shoulder Strike can help you develop the six connections, as there is very little external motion in the arms on the second phase of the movement.

During the first phase, as you close, sink your qi from

> shoulder to hip,
>> elbow to knee, and
>>> hand to foot.

Dropping your qi in this way connects up the body.

During the opening phase, the body moves as one piece, like a wall driven forward by a hydraulic ram. The power is expressed through the shoulder.

Without these connections:

the body moves top heavy;

the shoulder advances too far;

the wall crumbles and breaks; and

unification and power are lost!

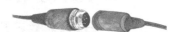

Six-pin plug – when the six pins align and slot into their sockets, energy can pass through

In Shoulder Strike:

The front foot, knee, hip, shoulder, elbow and hand are represented by the wall.

Using the weight shift from Principle 12, the back leg becomes the hydraulic ram, which drives the body forward.

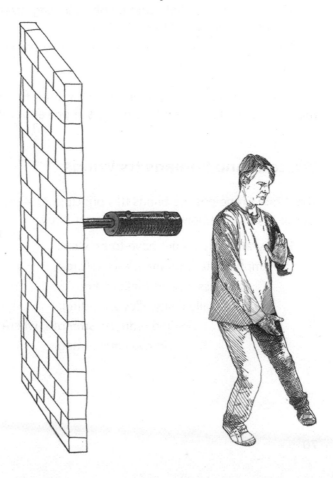

Principle 24:

Tune in to Heaven Above and Earth Below

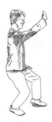

The heavens are light and open, manifesting the quality of expanding, yang energy.

Earth is heavy and full, manifesting the quality of condensing, yin energy.

These representations are reflected in the fundamental state of the body during all tai chi and qi gong practice:

> The upper body is light and empty, allowing power and strength to drain down to the lower half.

> The lower body is full and heavy, receiving the energy of the upper half.

In this way, the lower body supports and carries the upper body, while the upper body follows and expresses the power developed in the legs.

White Crane Spreads Its Wings

The White Crane posture brings this principle to life with its low, rooted stance and soft, supple and empty upper body.

> Empty and soft do not have to be weak:
> emptying tension manifests softness;
> softness creates malleability;
> malleability allows yielding;
> yielding redirects strength, where
> yin overcomes yang.

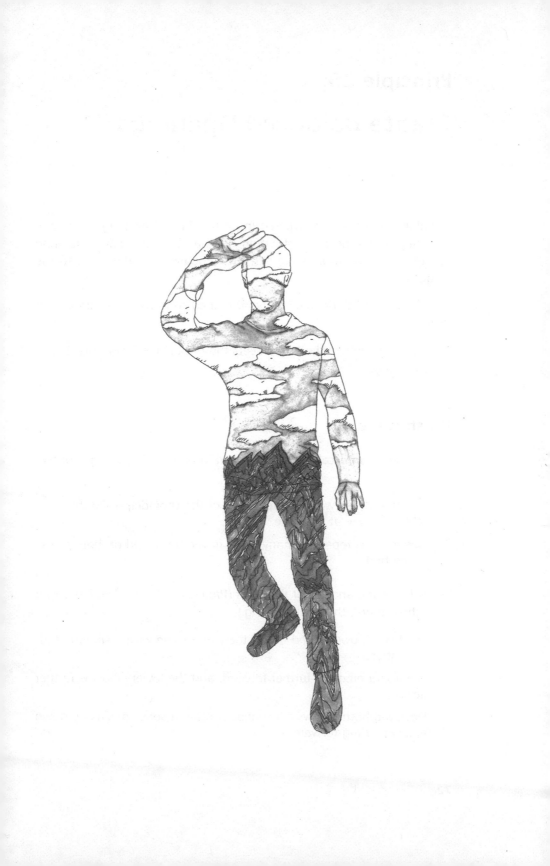

Principle 25:

Create Balanced Openings

A balanced opening is required in all tai chi and qi gong postures – whether symmetrical or not. Often one hand is further forward than the other, yet both arms are stretched equally from the spine to the fingertips.

This is achieved through careful and refined control of three important points:

> The spine, where the torso meets the neck (T1–C7 vertebrae).
>
> Both elbows.

Brush Knee

Brush Knee is an excellent posture to train balanced openings, for two reasons:

> One hand is forward at the height of the shoulder, while the other is lower, at the knee.
>
> This move is repeated many times in the form, and on both sides of the body.

The spine is the anchor for the arms (Principle 20), so T1–C7 rise ever so slightly during the final opening.

> The two elbows extend out of the rising spine with a smooth and even stretch.
>
> The upper elbow is further forward, and the lower elbow is further down.
>
> However, both elbows and hands contain a sense of sinking down and extending forward.

Together, these three firm yet sung forces create a balanced and equal opening without causing strain. When executed correctly, all three points separate evenly, which generates more internal space and, thereby, supports the mind sinking deeper into the body.

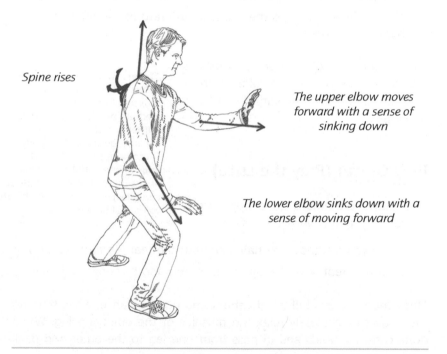

Spine rises

The upper elbow moves forward with a sense of sinking down

The lower elbow sinks down with a sense of moving forward

Principle 26:

The Continuum
of Empty versus Full

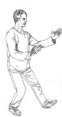

When shifting weight, the shift should be complete so as to leave one leg feeling "empty" and the other feeling "full".

This shifting allows for one leg to take the weight of the body while the other relaxes completely. In this way, the legs act like a pump that circulates blood and qi powerfully throughout the body.

The full leg receives the sinking fluids and roots your qi.

The empty leg receives the rising qi and returns the fluids back to the torso.

This continuum of motion strengthens the legs, opens the vascular system, circulates blood and interstitial fluid* and develops qi.

> *Interstitial fluid** is located between layers of soft-tissue cells and fibres, and is a medium by which cells receive nutrients and expel waste. On average the human body contains approximately 10 litres of interstitial fluid (more or less depending on individual variables) – more than double the volume of blood!

Play Guitar (Play the Lute)

Play Guitar presents a good opportunity to play with empty versus full, since:

when you advance, you half-step with the rear leg forward; and,

as you retreat, you pick up the front leg and put down the heel.

This action requires full weight shifts and good balance, while training the body to completely relax the muscles of the emptying leg. When done correctly, fluids and qi pass from one leg to the other and back again, like pouring water from one glass to another.

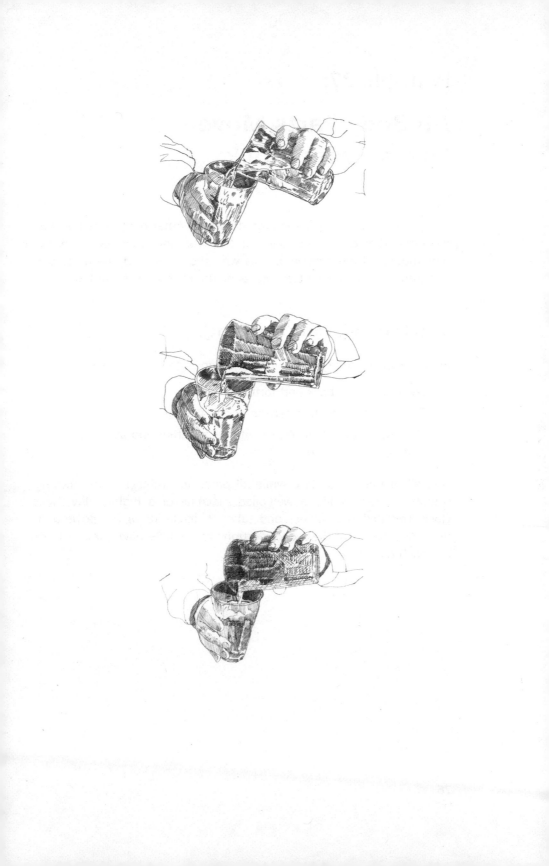

Principle 27:

All Body Parts Move Like a Swiss Clock

Every part of the body is integrated with all other parts, whether they move together, opposite to one another or in any other way. So if one part moves, all parts move. In this way, the entire body becomes one integrated whole, without any parts being left out of the motion.

Step Forward, Parry and Punch

In Step Forward, Parry and Punch, a complex tai chi movement:

> The body turns back and forth.
>
> The legs step and transfer the body's weight.
>
> The arms move in circles, sometimes together and at other times in opposite directions.

And all of this takes place while all parts are connected and moving smoothly together, like a well-oiled machine or a high-quality Swiss clock. This action combines and takes Principle 18 of the powertrain and Principle 23 of the six connections to a whole new level, so practise each diligently.

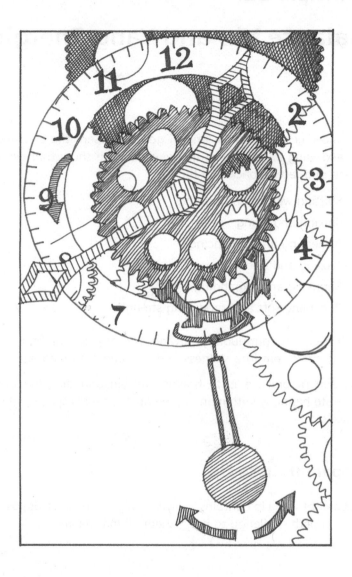

Principle 28:

Balance Yin and Yang Energies

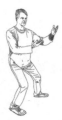 The movements of tai chi and qi gong represent the ebb and flow of yin and yang energies, like the waves on the shore that climb up the beach and recede back into the sea:

Shifting weight and turning.

Sinking and rising.

Retreating and advancing.

Closing and opening.

Shrinking and expanding.

Becoming soft and producing strength.

Each aspect is continuously flowing, like day into night, summer into winter, movement into stillness and circulation into storage.

The aim of practice is to balance all yin and all yang energies to generate harmony within and arrive at "the tai chi space", where peace prevails.

Apparent Close Up

Apparent Close Up contains a myriad of yin and yang opposites, offering a superb challenge to bring them all into balance.

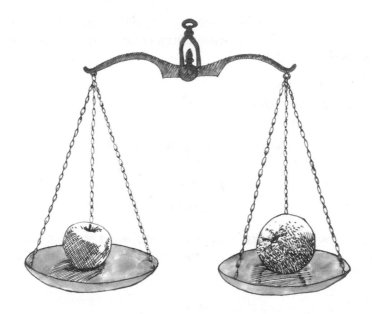

Principle 29:

The Body Moves in Circles

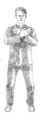

As in the natural order of the cosmos, all components of tai chi and qi gong movements are derived from circles – not straight lines. These can be expressed as:

Whole circles

Partial circles

Ellipses

Gentle and long curves or arcs

Loops

Teeny-tiny circles

Spirals

So all moves are circular in nature and avoid straight lines, because straight lines create inertia – the opponent of all internal arts, health and longevity.

Cross Hands

Cross Hands is built out of large, obvious circles on all three planes of motion, which allows even the most inexperienced student to get a taste of circularity. The advanced practitioner continues to train and hone even the most obvious techniques, for it is the refinement of the big that gives access to the small and subtle.

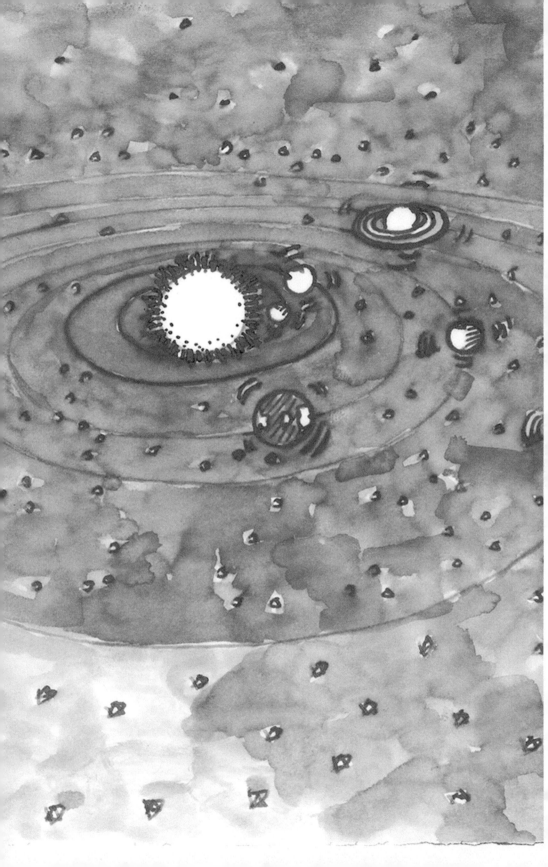

PART 3

Deeper Principles
for Fluidity and
Energy Development

Principle 30:

Generate Internal Momentum

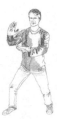

Water contained in a bath becomes disturbed when suddenly stirred with a wooden spoon. However, if you continue stirring in circles, slowly, smoothly, evenly and deliberately, eventually all of the water will move in unison with the stirring action.

Tai chi and qi gong forms engage and move blood and qi in a similar fashion, requiring slow, smooth, even and continuous motion with just the right quality:

without stops and starts;

without speeding up or slowing down.

To improve results, all excess tension needs to be released too. The smooth, continuous action helps to relax the body and nerves, and thus expels superficial and deeper tensions.

The longer you practise, the stronger the process becomes, and the more fully you engage the vascular system and qi flow – although never to the point of diminishing returns.

Embrace the Tiger, Return to the Mountain

The Embrace the Tiger, Return to the Mountain section of the form brings together various movements previously covered, with small additions and variations. This repetition allows the mind to deeply penetrate the body and develop the finesse required to generate internal momentum.

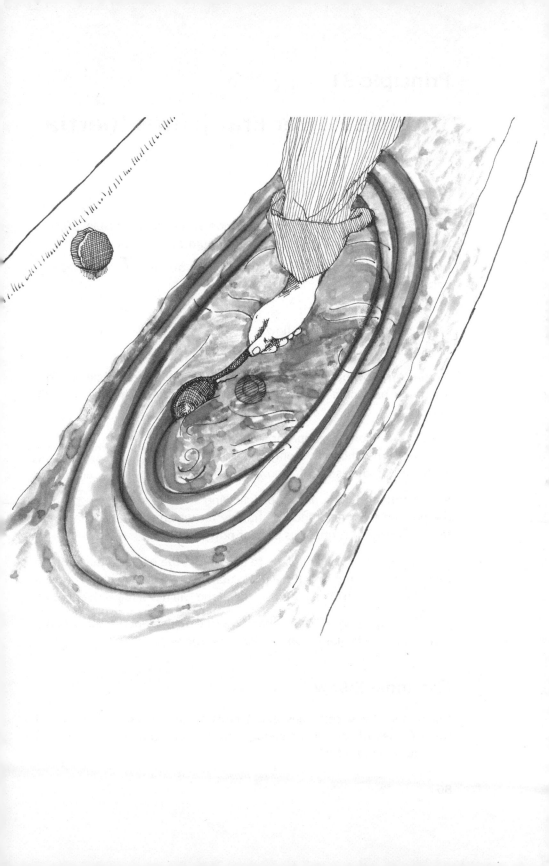

Principle 31:

Turbine Power Eradicates Inertia

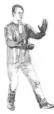

Once you have generated internal momentum via Principle 30, the next step is to use momentum in continuum to eradicate inertia.

Inertia is the enemy of internal arts training and living spontaneously, because it:

> Breaks momentum.
>
> Weakens blood and qi flow.
>
> Creates stagnation in body, mind and qi.

Inertia can show up in the form of a locked limb, tense muscle, motionless body part or a break in the flow, which diminishes whole-body motion.

Once in motion, a propeller engine or turbine* turns smoothly, evenly and effortlessly and produces thrust – *power*.

> *Propeller or turbine engines are rotary mechanical devices that convert fuel into continuous propulsive force.

So the turbine is one aspect of following the path of least resistance, a strategy for which the internal arts are famous, creating continuous circular power.

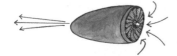

For an airplane to take flight, the engines must remain running. If the pilot cuts the power to the engines every 100 metres or so, the plane will never leave the ground.

Tai chi and qi gong utilise this principle to eradicate inertia through the continuum of circular motion within their forms.

Fist under Elbow

Fist under Elbow combines and blends large circular actions on all three planes of motion to engage the turbine and more powerfully circulate blood and qi.

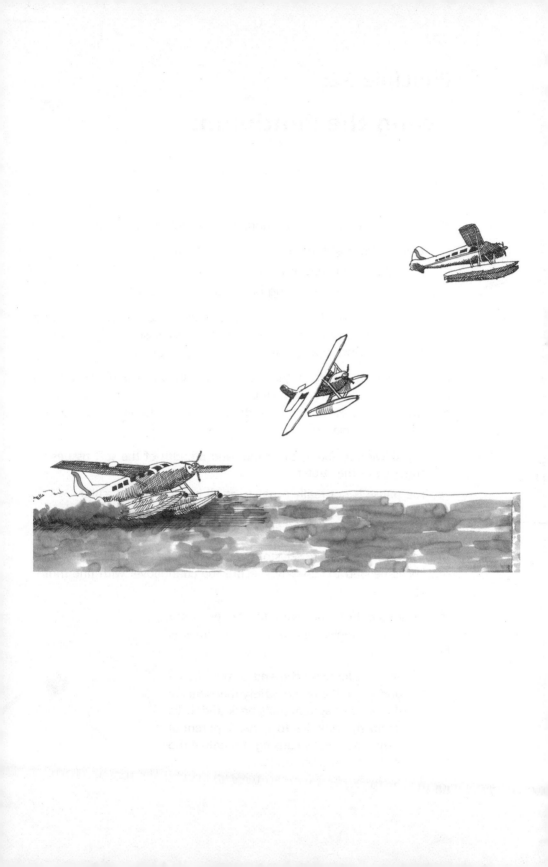

Principle 32:

Swing the Pendulum

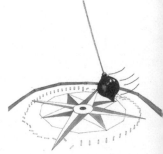

Study a large pendulum in motion, and you will notice that:

> it slows down at the end of its swing, then
> > momentarily pauses, before
> > > smoothly returning back from where it came.

This action is essential to internal arts training because, when reaching the end of any posture, the stretch in the soft tissues also comes to completion and the changeover mimics the pendulum.

Practise slowing down at the end of any stretches and allow for a momentary pause (but not a stop) before once again letting the fibres of your soft tissues return to neutral. All of this happens before you stretch into the next posture.

> The slowing is due to the depth and breadth of the soft tissues engaged in the stretch.

> The pause is not really a pause at all but, rather, a circular changeover from the extension to allow the fibres to begin the process of naturally and slowly returning to neutral.

In this way, the body never stops moving yet has the necessary time and focus needed to correctly execute the changeover with fine motor control.

If you stretch fast and hard to the end and begin the next move, one of two outcomes is likely to occur:

1. You suddenly hit the end of the stretch and ignite the body's safety mechanism; the nervous system pulls back and locks down the muscles to prevent potential damage, thereby causing a break in the flow. So you disconnect.

2. You quickly release the stretch, and the tissues snap back, like an elastic band snapping back to neutral after suddenly being released from a stretched-out position. So you also disconnect.

Disconnection generates inertia.

However, if you implement the pendulum swing inside your soft tissues while adhering to the Rule of Thirds:

The body softens and the nerves release.

Blood is pumped to the extremities and drawn back to the heart.

Qi extends out of the body and is drawn back in.

The space where yang and yin are balanced opens up.

The mind drops into a calm, peaceful state.

Repulse Monkey

Repulse Monkey is an excellent posture to engage the pendulum motion because, in the main aspect of the move, the two hands are like pendulums swinging in opposite directions. The posture is repeated several times and on each side of the body.

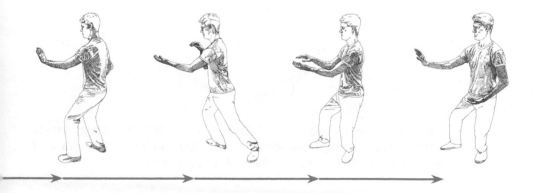

Principle 33:

Spring the Five Bows

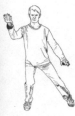

The five bows are:

Two arms

Two legs

Torso

The aim of bowing is to spring the arms and legs off the spine, the way a bow springs as the cord is drawn back and released.

Both the load and release are deliberate and slow to prevent building tension while storing and releasing power.

The four limbs connect to and are driven by the spine, which is an essential connection required to generate whole-body motion.

This is the fundamental process. However, there's more ...

A four-beat cycle guides the store-and-release process:

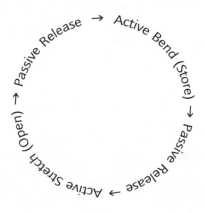

This continuous cycling — active bend, passive release, active stretch, passing release — embeds a sense of perpetual motion in the form, and the path of least resistance unfolds of its own accord.

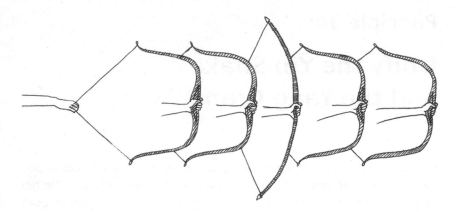

Slanted Flying

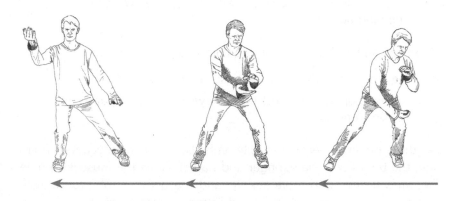

Slanted Flying is a superb posture for training and activating the five bows in total unison, as the body sinks low to bend and store, and stretches out to the extremities during the release and open.

Principle 34:

Unify the Yin Snake and the Yang Crane

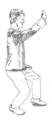

Legend has it that Shang San Feng, the founder of tai chi, developed the art after watching a fight between a snake and a crane. Whether fact or fiction, the movements of tai chi blend the qualities of both creatures.

> The yin aspect is the snake, with its powerful, pulsing, coiling action.

> The yang aspect is the crane, with its graceful, wave-like, whipping action.

The two combine to form a strong core and a soft exterior.

> The core becomes strong because yin energy condenses.

> The exterior becomes soft because yang energy expands and releases tension.

As these qualities become deeply embodied over some years of training, the bones become stronger and harder, while the muscular frame becomes flexible and more supple, and the body morphs to produce the quality of an iron bar wrapped in many layers of cloth – strength cloaked in softness.

White Crane Spreads Its Wings

All tai chi seeks to further the embodiment of the fundamental balancing act of yin and yang energies. White Crane Spreads Its Wings is a natural point in the form to begin this aspect of your journey.

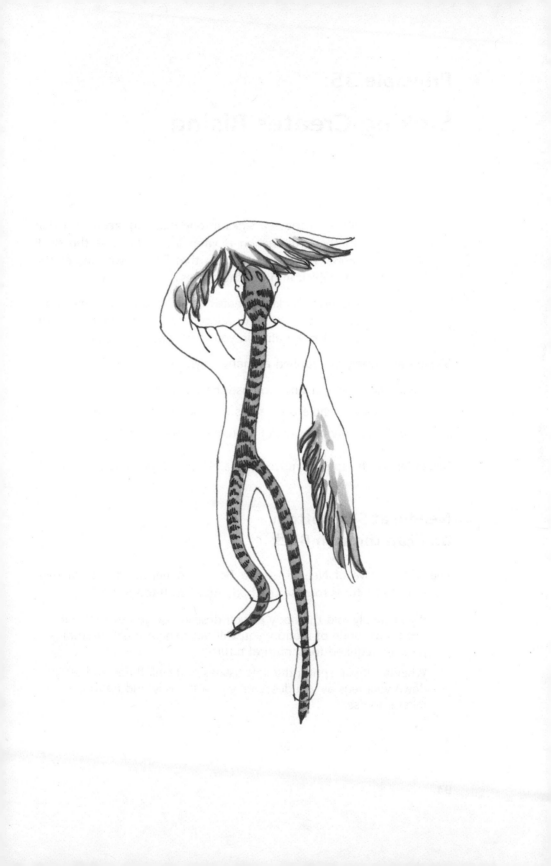

Principle 35:

Sinking Creates Rising

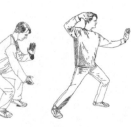

Water in the sea sinks in one place to create a rise in another. This action is what lifts a boat as the swell grows. Principle 14 states that "the down creates the up", which initiates the process.

Likewise, "sinking creates rising" is a deeper and more profound internal development, which requires Principle 14 to be alive in your flesh and a sung body.

Sinking and rising are applied in many ways:

Sometimes one arm sinks to raise the other.

Sometimes the whole body sinks to raise one or both arms.

Other times only the sinking shoulders raise the arms.

Regardless of the specific movement, sinking always creates rising.

Needle at Sea Bottom and Fan through Back

The whole move of Needle at Sea Bottom generates the downward pressure that returns to raise the body into Fan through Back.

If you simply fold the body as you descend or go beyond your two-thirds range of motion, you will not generate the internal pressure required for a natural return.

Whereas, if you spring the soft tissues and sink fluids and qi down your legs as you descend, you will easily and naturally release to rise.

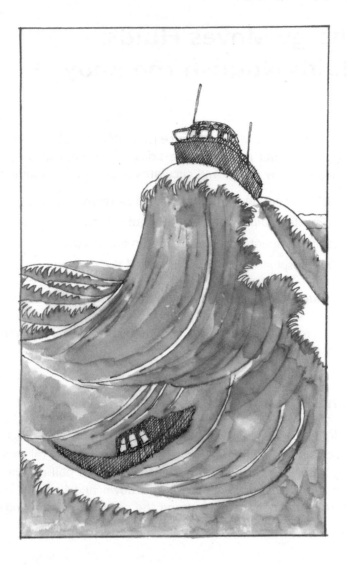

Principle 36:

Energy Moves Fluids, Fluids Nourish the Body

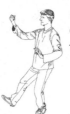 Like the moon's gravitational force (potential energy) moves the waters of the ocean and influences the tides, the movement of qi energy in the human body moves and circulates bodily fluids, including:

Blood – contained within the cardiovascular system.

Interstitial fluid – between layers of soft-tissue cells and fibres.

Lymph – an integral part of the immune system.

Cerebrospinal fluid – in and around the brain, and spinal cord.

These fluids flush out toxins, metabolic waste and dead material and replace them with nutrients that allow the body to grow, repair and thrive. Circulating bodily fluids is one of the secrets of Water method longevity practices.

Turn and Chop with the Fist

Moving qi, blood and other bodily fluids is fundamental to Water method arts training in all forms; however, Yang style tai chi's Turn and Chop with the Fist uses large sagittal circles to pull qi (and therefore draws the fluids) down and up, and down and back up the body – strengthening qi flow and bathing the cells in life-sustaining nutrients.

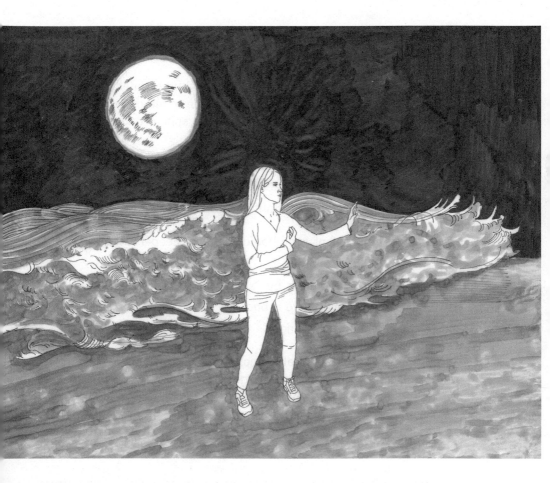

Principle 37:

Balance the Sphere

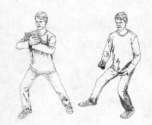 The sphere refines and develops three-dimensional circular movement by unifying it into one coherent whole. Blending and integrating circles into the sphere takes place on all three planes of motion:

Transverse – horizontal

Sagittal – front-back vertical

Coronal – left-right vertical

As spherical movement is embodied on ever deeper levels, all motion follows one simple rule:

if there is down, there is up;

if there is forward, there is back;

if there is left, there is right.

This is not done sequentially, one after the other, but in the same moment, all together: the body begins to shrink and grow in all directions simultaneously in a balanced and harmonious way.

Lu and Ji

Building on Principle 19, Soften to Close, Release to Open, the postures of Lu and Ji exemplify pure yin and pure yang, respectively.

Lu absorbs as it condenses – without contraction.

Ji projects as it expands – without strain.

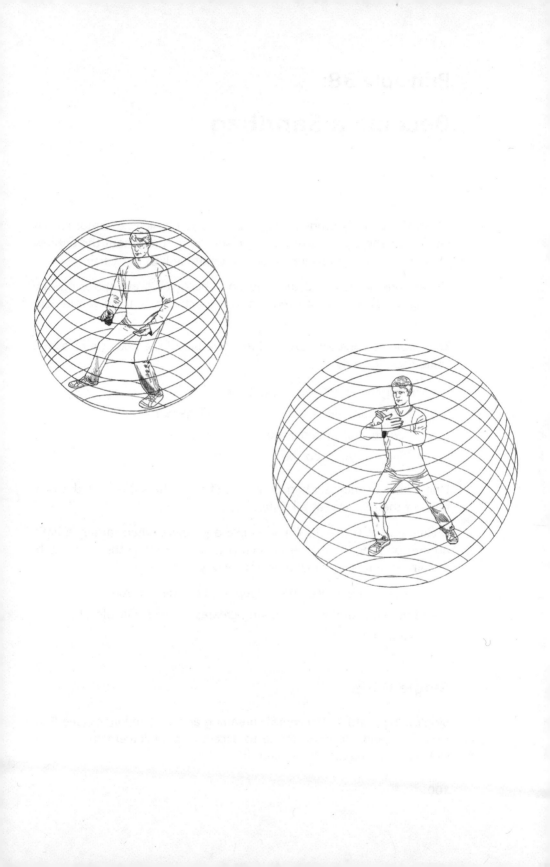

Principle 38:

Become a Sandbag

When the body is properly aligned and the physical, external root is well established, you naturally begin sinking qi throughout the entirety of your form. This cultivates a more intimate link to the Earth.

As tensions are released and the body becomes ever-more sung, the sinking drives deeper into your body and activates sinking within your insides.

The whole rib cage and external musculature of the body drops as the spine rises upwards.

> The organs sink down in the torso;
>> the fluids sink down through the legs to the feet;
>>> qi sinks deeper into the earth, and
>>>> your root becomes internal.

One corner of the sandbag is always lifted – the spine. But the contents of the bag sink at all times.

Building on Principle 15 (moving like a puppet), when raising a limb, an arm or a leg, it is done in such a way as to allow the contents to remain continuously sinking. In this way, you develop:

> Exceptional balance and a deep, well-established root.
> Continuous qi flow via "sinking creates rising" (Principle 35).
> A calm mind.

Single Whip

Single Whip, with its horizontal spreading action of the limbs (see Principle 21), yields an open frame to access and implement the internal sinking of the organs, fluids and qi.

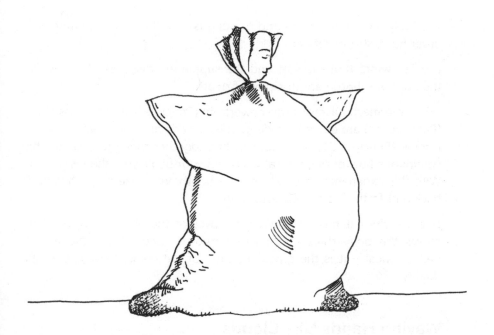

Principle 39:

Ride the Wave

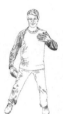

The body motion in tai chi and qi gong is soft, fluid and continuous – never hard, stiff or robotic.

Lao Tzu wrote that the soft and the supple are disciples of life, while the hard and brittle are disciples of death.[18]

When the mechanisms of the powertrain (Principle 18) and Swiss clock (Principle 27) are embedded deep in your body and the function of the turbine (Principle 31) is brought to life, together they give way to the continuous flow of qi, physically moving your body from the inside out. With this experience, you will feel a smooth, wave-like force that runs back and forth throughout your flesh.

Like a surfer catches and rides the waves of the ocean, a wave of qi moves the body through three-dimensional space. The wave is not metaphorical – it is the graceful action of the crane, fully alive in its fluidity.

Waving Hands Like Clouds

Waving Hands Like Clouds generates this graceful, wave-like action, softening deeper and deeper layers of your mind-body-qi matrix. The form is circular, fluid and repetitive, giving you the opportunity to feel, follow and ride the wave.

Empty the body of resistance,
and your body will fill with qi.

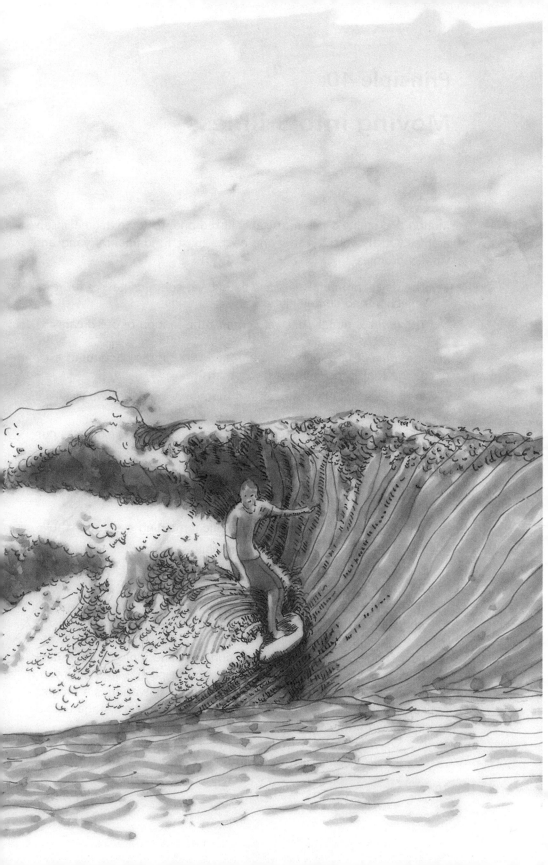

Principle 40:

Moving into Stillness

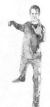

Motion and stillness are inextricably linked and, to some degree, inseparable. Activity versus rest is one of the most fundamental yang and yin dichotomies.

The day is primarily an active period, yet contains pauses for rest, reflection and contemplation.

The night is mainly still, yet contains the motion of our dreams.

The interplay of opposites sets the framework for the continuous cycle of change that living a life involves, both

in the external environment and the planet on which we live, as well as

within ourselves, our internal world, as each of us experiences our Self.

The macrocosm and microcosm are one, so to understand that which is outside, look inside:

In **body**, seek fluid, free motion while remaining even and stable.

In **qi**, seek flow and amplification while storing what you develop.

In **emotions**, seek neutrality and balance while allowing them to be smooth and unsuppressed.

In **mind**, seek calmness and presence as the guiding force of the body and its qi.

Merging stillness in motion and motion in stillness plagues the dedicated practitioner until they realise that both aspects – in their myriad combinations – paradoxically coexist together. Cultivation is a progressive, cyclical process (as covered in Principle 1), with each stage unfolding in its own time.

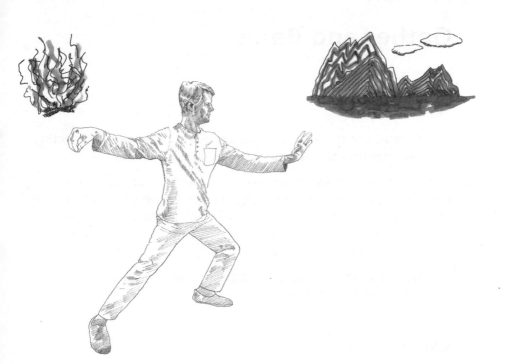

Single Whip

The last Single Whip in this section of the form is an ideal point to practise moving into stillness during motion. Continue this training through the many cycles of your practice to lead yourself into your core knowing that, in order to fully realise its potential, this principle relies upon Principle 21, Opposites Spread Open the Body, and Principle 38, Become a Sandbag, previously covered by Single Whip.

Principle 41:

Gather and Bank

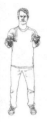

The last action of the form is to gather your qi and bank it for another time, whether later that day or at some point in the future.

Begin by decreasing your effort, giving less and less to each part of the move without dramatically reducing the size of the external form. All internal aspects and qi flows you have managed to ignite are already up and running, and now it's time to take the foot off the throttle and coast downhill to your destination.

> Ease off slowly, not suddenly. Breaking the flow causes inertia and, thereby, stagnation.

Closing Form

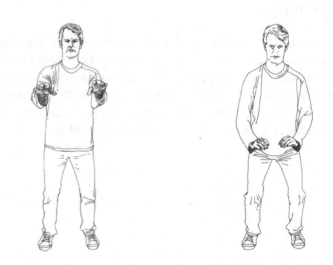

Closing Form is exactly that – closing the form. It's basically the same externally as Beginning Form, except you are not warming and opening up the body, but instead preparing for rest.

The final act is to softly, smoothly and evenly expand your body, including:

    All of your tissues.
    All of your fluids.
    All of your qi.

Then, smoothly, gently and slowly let your body return to neutral using the capillary action that has been generated by the release to draw blood back into the organs and qi into the lower tantien.

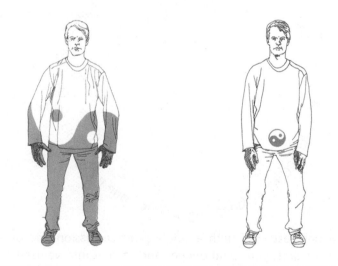

Principle 42:

Postures Link into Fluid Forms

All postures in tai chi and qi gong forms link together to create continuous, fluid motion. There is no stop or break at any point.

When achieved, the energy generated in one movement is successfully passed on to the next one in the chain, and the synergy builds exponentially.

> This is what is meant in *The Tai Chi Classics* by:
> "From posture to posture internal energy remains unbroken."[19]

The momentum generated and maintained, from beginning to end, can produce sublime and profound results.

Of course, all principles and aspects of learning are also linked, woven, balanced and unified within the form.

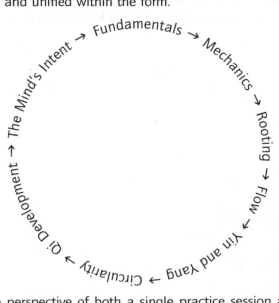

From the perspective of both a single practice session and of regular practice over time, you spiral deeper and deeper into yourself, moving closer towards your core.

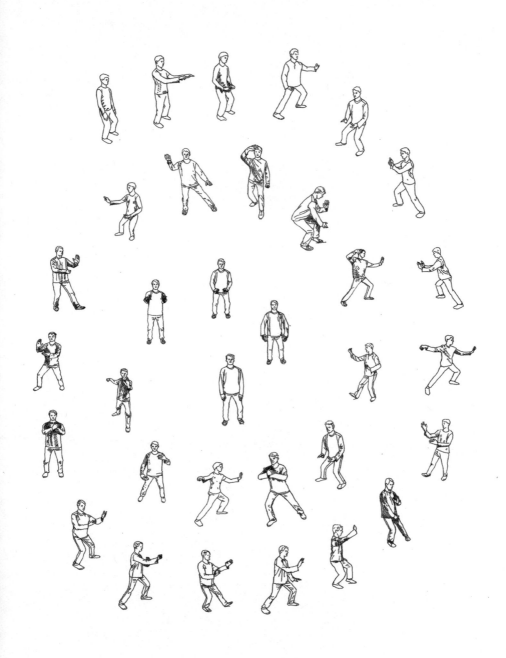

Afterword

"A journey of a thousand miles begins with a single step."

Taoist Sage Lao Tzu

The Water method is the root of internal principles as described by Lao Tzu in the classic text, the *Tao Te Ching*,[20] 2,500 years ago. This methodology encourages following the path of least resistance while learning strategies for yielding to and blending with nature, and the one constant in life – change.

Water method energy arts mimic the properties of water, which, when flowing, is fresh, free and alive.

More flow begets less resistance.

Less resistance begets less tension.

Less tension begets more naturalness.

The more natural you are, the closer you move towards your core.

The act of moving towards your core is precisely what allows your true path to unfold.

Internal energy arts training makes this possible because, through systematic and progressive techniques, it weaves together the various threads that make up all aspects of ourselves* and unifies the seemingly paradoxical differences within us into one whole and balanced human being.

*For example, the body, energy, emotions, mind and spirit of any individual.

So how can you get started on this momentous journey? It is the principles of tai chi and qi gong that first build your foundation and then, over time, guide development of your Self from the inside out.

Blood and Qi Are Inseparable

Water method training is pragmatic and always begins with the body; it next moves through the realms of qi and integrates the two at the level of the mind.

If blood moves, qi moves.

If qi moves, blood moves.

The horse and cart are intimately connected; therefore, if the cart moves, the horse must move too. But the ideal scenario is, of course, for the horse to pull the cart; that is, for *qi to move blood*.

In the internal arts, the aim is to make contact with and unify your qi with your mind; this is how you gain control of your blood flow, which is a key to developing health, vitality and power for healing, longevity and self-defence Your intent is the mechanism through which you achieve this unity, a skill, and which decisively puts the mind in the driving seat – in charge of the horse.

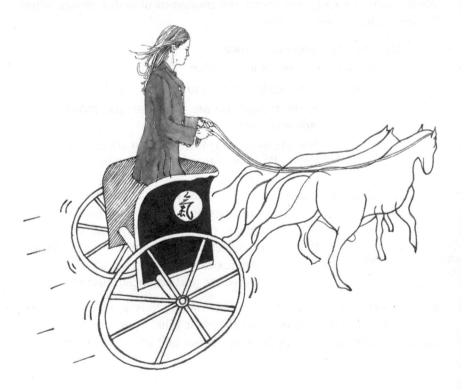

The mind contacts and mobilises qi to amplify the healing and power-generating faculties of the internal arts.

Qi grabs the blood and generates more powerful circulation.

Blood circulation activates the soft tissues and sets the body into motion.

When the body is firmly on its healing journey, from having cleared a reasonable amount of the tension that resided there, a rebalancing is initiated and a positive feedback loop that fine-tunes the mind is enacted. Yes, brain function is upgraded, but so too is your ability to see yourself and the world through new eyes: perception of Self and your environment changes, which can also change your relationship to and your place within your environment. The process of self-development naturally trends towards the empathic, compassionate and, perhaps, even spiritual.*

*Spiritual does not necessarily mean religious, although religion may or may not come into play for an individual.

Spiritual, in the realm of internal arts, is about cultivation of spirit – or a higher vibration of energy than the mundane qi needed to operate and keep your body healthy. The Water method regards everything in the universe as energy, vibrating at different frequencies and resonating according to that to which it is attuned. Studying the nature of Self – what you are attuned to – is what allows you to enter the game of self-discovery and break through your conditioning to become free from externally imposed rules and walk your own path.

The ancients designed and meticulously refined internal energy arts over millennia so that any individual who puts in some measure of time, effort and reasonably clear intent to their practice could naturally progress to the next level,* to gain deeper understanding – hence the quote attributed to Lao Tzu of a journey starting with a single step, which enables the next, and so on. The internal principles are the steps that systematically guide practice and cultivation of Self.

*This is not to say that live training from a competent and willing teacher is not necessary. On the contrary, there is very little chance for any student – no matter how talented – to access the deeper and more subtle aspects of internal arts training without an experienced teacher, especially relating to the higher realms of self-development.

The Fabric of the Internal Arts

In the beginning, the gross or obvious meanings of the principles come to light to get you on your way. At this stage, not all aspects of all principles presented here will be continuously active. And you certainly do not want to try to make it so, as the mind will simply play the juggler – rapidly and sequentially cycling through principles, which not only leads to purely mental processing, but also undermines cohesion and integration of internal techniques and, more importantly, of Self.

As you focus on and systematically begin to embody principles, one by one, each remains active as you move on to the next. And, indeed, this is your rule of measure: when you focus your mind's intent on one principle while other threads you have previously trained remain active, you know you have actually integrated them. If they weaken or fall away, you know they need more attention. Some principles may come online for you relatively quickly, whereas others might require many more weeks, months or even years of practice to honestly achieve any depth and range of skill and application.

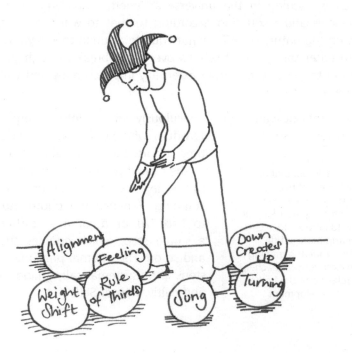

As you embody ever more threads of internal techniques that weave together and give shape to your forms, you also become aware of the holes in your skill set. Not to worry, as they provide direction for your practice. In a high-quality cloth, you will not find blemishes or clumps of thread, and the same is true for the fabric of the internal arts. Seek out errors, then adjust, refine and hone your art into a seamless integration of external form and internal content.

All change, all healing and the creative force takes place in the here and now. So when it comes to practice, approach yourself as a human being instead of a human doing: that is, as something that must be improved or overcome, and in a set time frame too.

Practicalities

The Yang style postures presented in this text are derived from the form of Yang Cheng Fu, a direct descendant of the Yang family, as I consider it to be a superb balance between ease of learning and depth of internals; however, internal principles can be applied to any tai chi or qi gong form.

Why Stop at Waving Hands Like Clouds?

After Waving Hands Like Clouds comes the Kick Section of the form, where most students lose their balance and, more importantly, their internal connection. When balance is lost, the muscles tighten to prevent toppling over, and the mind is thrown out of the body in order to heighten awareness of its surroundings. When this happens, all of the goodness that has been developed throughout your form suddenly goes out the window. So until you have a firm grasp on the beginning sections of the form and can maintain physical balance *and* internal connections while on one leg, it is most likely counterproductive to continue further into the form.

In the beginning, there were only Long Forms because the ancient Chinese had plenty of time and space to practise. Over time, many masters began passing down shorter forms for ease of learning and to make the arts available to a wider population. Some teachers use the First Section of their Long Form as a Short Form, whereas others use Grasp the Bird's Tail up to the first Single Whip as a Mini Form. Personally, I find up to the first Waving Hands Like Clouds a good balance between the time needed to generate strong circulation and develop qi, yet short enough to fit into people's busy schedules and physical space. You can simply repeat the form for as many rounds as you can remain relaxed and present, and steer clear of diminishing returns.

There are many more complex movements in the form after Waving Hands Like Clouds – not just the kicks – but also more demanding postures, such as Snake Creeps Down and Fair Lady Weaves the Shuttles. Few Westerners can correctly execute these postures without inducing tension or grossly overshooting the Rule of Thirds. So the wise tai chi student focuses on opening, releasing tension from and strengthening their body before adding to complexity or physical demands. Muscles need to become soft and loose, and you require a good sense of your physical abilities and limitations. After all, being honest with yourself and facing the reality of where you are in the here and now is how you cultivate a healthy relationship with yourself and progress at the fastest rate. Minding the Rule of Thirds is the key to building health and vitality from the inside out – instead of from the demands of the ego, which pushes you beyond your comfortable limits ... just to look good in the park!

Repeat Moves

Some of the repeated moves in the form, such as the second Raise Hands, Step Forward, Parry and Punch as well as several repetitions of An, were intentionally left out. These postures, along with the principles they carry, are covered in the first section of the form and, due to their importance, require copious practice. There is nothing more to add at this level of the game, and simply layering in more techniques to satisfy the drive for new! new! new! undermines rather than improves skill.

Layering

Other repeated moves, such as Single Whip and White Crane Spreads Its Wings, contain a new principle each time they are visited. This is because the principles build on each other and the principle shown on the first round must be deeply embodied in your flesh to truly experience the second- and, in the case of Single Whip, even third-level principle. In most cases, the more fundamental principle is presented in the first section of the form with the higher and more advanced principle in the second. This is the case with Lu and Ji, which contain Soften to Close, Release to Open (Principle 19) in the first section and Balance the Sphere (Principle 37) in the second. However, there are other layers, such as the Powertrain (Principle 18), which is the foundation for All Body Parts Move Like a Swiss Clock (Principle 27) – both are in the first section.

These are some of the more obvious progressions, but if you devote time and effort to learning principles and practising them, you will discover many more connections and feedback loops. More advanced principles also refine all previous principles, and the whole cycle of practice begins again. The inescapable circular nature of training is how all of the various threads are woven together and either directly or indirectly link to all others to create one fabric. It is the weave that accounts for the strength and quality of the cloth, not any single thread.

To Advance, First Retreat

Internal energy arts are diverse and multi-layered, offering the potential to develop all aspects of yourself. As your needs change, there is no necessity to look externally to find new forms or practices. Instead, the focus of your mind's intent and your training changes to yield the desired result. The principles of tai chi and qi gong ensure we walk a true path through the process. They are designed in such a way as to allow students who adhere to their ancient wisdom to learn and progressively hone their skill set, while tuning in to ever-deeper subtleties of training.

Principle 42, the last one, covers how postures link together into one balanced and coherent form. But a chain is only as strong as the weakest links, so again this is why the Eastern mindset plays to weaknesses – so they can root them out and strengthen them!

Without balance, there is no integration.

Without integration, there is no whole, no unity.

Without unity, effort is wasted and results simply dissipate.

So if you have a genuine desire to take your practice to the moon, first get rooted here on Earth. Develop and refine each individual component you learn in addition to complete forms. Continue this strategy throughout every stage of your development, in all forms, leaving no stone unturned. The momentum you build in your practice will grow and multiply exponentially. In the realm of the internal arts, fluid, circular forms, which can only be generated by adhering to the fundamental principles, are what all dedicated practitioners aim to achieve. It is this seamless integration of form and content, the fusion of engineering and art, that systematically and progressively cultivates the energy to heal, become vibrant, apply power for martial arts and even follow a spiritual path, as you so choose.

Moving towards the Tai Chi Space

We live in a dualistic reality, where it is impossible to manifest only one side of a coin. You have two arms, two legs, two eyes and two ears, two lungs and two kidneys, two hemispheres of your brain and two opposing flows of blood in your body (via arteries and veins). We cannot experience day without night, activity without rest, or good without bad. These dichotomies permeate our flesh, qi and mind, and the entire natural world in which we live. Yet too many human beings make a mess of their realities because they do not acknowledge this simple fact. The mind always wants events to play out in a single, linear progression to fulfil even the most whimsical of desires. We want more of what we like and none of what we do not. But the simple fact remains that the manifest realm is always a blend of dualities, of yin and yang.

Tai chi or *tai ji* literally means "all oneness", referring to the state an adept experiences when all yins and all yangs have been balanced, harmonised and integrated within their body, mind and qi. This state opens up immense space within the consciousness of the adept who achieves this profound level of practice. The tai chi space is both the carrot one moves towards, as well as the destination that guides and gives shape to an individual's training. As you work through the 42 principles, practising, reflecting and refining them over time, your body will open, your qi will grow and your mind will morph, laying the essential foundation to move towards and enter into the tai chi space.

REFERENCES

1. Wayne, Peter M., PhD, with Mark L. Fuerst, *The Harvard Medical School Guide to Tai Chi*. Shambhala Publications, 2013.
2. *Cheng Man-ch'ing: Master of Five Excellences*, translated by Mark Hennessy. Frog Books, an imprint of North Atlantic Books, 1995.
   Olson, Stuart Alve, *Steal My Art: The Life and Times of T'ai Chi Master T.T. Liang*. North Atlantic Books, 2002.
3. Frantzis, Bruce, *The Power of Internal Martial Arts and Chi*, pp. 350–351. Blue Snake Books, an imprint of North Atlantic Books, 1998, 2007.
4. Lao Tzu, *Tao Te Ching: The Definitive Edition*, translated by Jonathan Star, p. 3. Penguin Group, 2001.
5. Frantzis, Bruce, *Opening the Energy Gates of Your Body*, pp. 89–90. Energy Arts, Inc. and North Atlantic Books, 1993, 2006.
6. Kaptchuk, Ted J., *The Web That Has No Weaver: Understanding Chinese Medicine*, pp. 62–65. Congdon and Weed, Inc., 1983.
7. Watts, Alan, "The Nature of Consciousness", 1960 article, https://erowid.org/culture/characters/watts_alan/watts_alan_article1.shtml
8. Davis, Barbara, *The Taijiquan Classics: An Annotated Translation*. Blue Snake Books, an imprint of North Atlantic Books, Inc., 2004.
   Lee, Ying-arng, *Lee's Modified Tai Chi Chuan for Health*. Unicorn Press, 1974.
9. Lao Tzu, *Tao Te Ching: The Definitive Edition*, translated by Jonathan Star. Penguin Books Ltd, 2001.
10. *I Ching or Book of Changes:* The Richard Wilhelm Translation by Cary F. Baynes. Bollingen Foundation, 1950.
    Ritsema, Rudolf and Sabbadini, Shantena Augusto, *The Original I Ching Oracle: The Pure and Complete texts with Concordance*. Watkins Publishing Group, Inc., 2005.
11. Chuang Tzu, *The Book of Chuang Tzu*, translated by Martin Palmer. Penguin Books Ltd, 1996.
    Zhuangzi (Chuang Tzu) *Zhuangzi: Basic Writings*, translated by Burton Watson. Columbia University Press, 2003.

12. Chuang Tzu, *The Way of Chuang Tzu*, translated by Thomas Merton. Shambhala Publications, 2004.

13. *Chuang-Tzu: The Inner Chapters*. Hackett Publishing Company, Inc., 2001.

14. Netter, Frank H., MD, *Atlas of Human Anatomy: Fourth Edition*. Saunders, an imprint of Saunders, 1989, 1997, 2003, 2006.

15. Netter, Frank H., MD, *Atlas of Human Anatomy: Fourth Edition*. Saunders, an imprint of Saunders, 1989, 1997, 2003, 2006.

16. Kuprenas, John, *101 Things I Learned in Engineering School*. Grand Central Publishing, 2013.

17. Lao Tzu, *Tao Te Ching: The Definitive Edition*, translated by Jonathan Star, Verse 11, p. 24. Penguin Books Ltd, 2001.

18. Tzu, Lao, *Tao Te Ching: The Definitive Edition*, translated by Jonathan Star, Verse 76, p. 89. Penguin Group, 2001.

19. This translation is the one used by Tai Chi Master Bruce Frantzis, who is fluent in Mandarin and studied with famous masters in China, Japan and Taiwan.

20. Lao Tzu, *Tao Te Ching: The Definitive Edition*, translated by Jonathan Star. Penguin Books Ltd, 2001.
    Lao Tzu, *Tao Te Ching*, translated by D.C Lau. Penguin Books Ltd, 1963.
    Lao Tzu, *Tao Te Ching*, translated by Stephen Addiss and Stanley Lombardo, p. 76. Hackett Publishing Company, Inc., 1993.

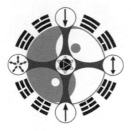

Paul Cavel is the founder of the London-based internal arts school,
The Tai Chi Space

He also offers seminars throughout Europe
and seasonal retreats in Andalusia, Spain

Correspondence address:

Paul Cavel
Kemp House
152 City Road
London EC1V 2NX
United Kingdom

+44 (0)7411 418 018

qi@paulcavel.com

www.PaulCavel.com